DATE DUE

NOV 22 '95			
DEC 20 1996			
APR 24 1999			
DEC 12 1999			
MAY 05 2000			
NOV 02 2000			
121302			
NOV 19 2003			
042104			
DEC 01 2005			
DEC 15 2009			

HIGHSMITH 45-220

ALCOHOL DISABILITIES PRIMER:

A GUIDE TO PHYSICAL AND PSYCHOSOCIAL DISABILITIES CAUSED BY ALCOHOL USE

Bozena-Eva Robertson, Ph.D.

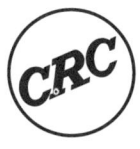

CRC Press
Boca Raton   Ann Arbor   London   Tokyo

Library of Congress Cataloging-in-Publication Data

Robertson, Bozena-Eva.
    Alcohol disabilities primer : a guide to physical and psychosocial disabilities caused by alcohol use / by Bozena-Eva Robertson.
    p.   cm.
    Includes bibliographical references and index.
    ISBN 0-8493-8966-6
    1. Alcoholism--Complications.   2. Alcoholism--Social aspects.
  I. Title.
    RC565.R63   1993
    616.86′1--dc20   93-22609
                                                                                                      CIP

    This book represents information obtained from authentic and highly regarded sources. Reprinted material is quoted with permission, and sources are indicated. A wide variety of references are listed. Every reasonable effort has been made to give reliable data and information, but the author and the publisher cannot assume responsibility for the validity of all materials or for the consequences of their use.

    Neither this book nor any part may be reproduced or transmitted in any form or by any means, electronic or mechanical, including photocopying, microfilming, and recording, or by any information storage and retrieval system, without permission in writing from the publisher.

    Direct all inquiries to CRC Press, Inc., 2000 Corporate Blvd., N.W., Boca Raton, Florida 33431.

© 1993 by CRC Press, Inc.

International Standard Book Number 0-8493-8966-6

Library of Congress Card Number 93-22609

Printed in the United States of America 1 2 3 4 5 6 7 8 9 0

Printed on acid-free paper

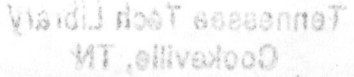

This book is dedicated to
Courtney and Mark Robertson.

PREFACE

During my doctoral studies at Syracuse University in the Rehabilitation Counseling Program, I had the good fortune of taking a course with Professor Michael Marge. The course dealt with the prevention of human disabilities. As Dr. Marge outlined the primary causes of disabilities, it became apparent to me that alcohol was implicated in all fifteen causes, many of which were completely preventable. The seeds of this project took root at that time.

Alcohol as a contributing factor to many physical and/or psychosocial complications became an integral part of several substance abuse counseling courses I was asked to teach by Dr. Ken Reagles at Syracuse University. What took seed in Dr. Marge's class, began to take on a clearer form and focus. Many of the existing texts pertaining to alcohol abuse merely touched upon the various debilitating consequences of chronic alcohol use. It was evident that to clearly present the breadth and depth of the consequences of chronic alcohol use, a separate text was needed; hence, the Alcohol Disabilities Primer.

Bozena-Eva Robertson, Ph.D.

THE AUTHOR

Bozena-Eva Robertson, Ph.D., is currently in private practice and working as a consultant in the Philadelphia area.

Dr. Robertson graduated in 1975 from the State University College of New York at Buffalo with a B.S.Ed. degree in art education. She obtained her M.S. degree in Rehabilitation Counseling in 1978 from the State University of New York at Buffalo. In 1989, Dr. Robertson received her Ph.D. degree in Rehabilitation Counseling from Syracuse University. She holds certifications both in rehabilitation counseling and school counseling.

Until 1991, Dr. Robertson served as an Adjunct Professor at Syracuse University (Syracuse, New York) where she taught courses in Counseling Theory, Rehabilitation Methods of Substance Abusers, Orientation to Substances of Abuse, and Rehabilitation of Psychiatrically Disabled Individuals. In 1990 and 1991, Dr. Robertson served as the Director of the Central New York Veterans Outreach Center in Syracuse, New York. 1992, she was asked to develop and implement the substance abuse program at the Rehabilitation Center of Philadelphia, a traumatic brain injury facility.

Dr. Robertson is a member of the American Counseling Association, American Rehabilitation Counseling Association, the National Rehabilitation Association, the National Rehabilitation Counselors Association, and the National Head Injury Foundation.

Dr. Robertson's current research interests are in survivors of emotional, physical and sexual abuse, and positive and negative coping strategies used by children and adults in dysfunctional families.

ACKNOWLEDGMENTS

It is with deep gratitude that I acknowledge the following individuals, without whom this book may not have come to fruition.

Michael Marge, Ed.D., Syracuse University, for providing the forum in which to illustrate how alcohol contributes to disabilities.

Kenneth Reagles, Ph.D., Syracuse University, mentor and advisor.

Roseann Falise, Ph.D., for her support, clarity and focus in the naming of this project.

Paul L. Petralia, Life Science Editor, for his support, interest, and enthusiasm in this endeavor.

A special note of thanks to my husband, Gary, who once again survived my many hours of obsessive and erratic behavior. His support and understanding was invaluable.

TABLE OF CONTENTS

Preface.................................. v

Acknowledgments........................viii

INTRODUCTION
   I.   ALCOHOL AND DISABILITIES....... 1
   II. PREVALENCE OF ALCOHOL ABUSE
        AND DEPENDENCE................. 5
   III. PREVENTION OF DISABILITIES..... 7

CHAPTER 1
ALCOHOL AND FETAL COMPLICATIONS........ 15
   I.   BIRTH DEFECTS.................. 15
   II. PERINATAL COMPLICATIONS........ 20

CHAPTER 2
ALCOHOL AND ACUTE OR CHRONIC ILLNESS.... 29
   I.   ACUTE AND CHRONIC ILLNESS...... 29

CHAPTER 3
ALCOHOL AND ADVERSE SOCIAL CONSEQUENCES. 59
   I.   ACCIDENTS...................... 59
       A. Traffic Accidents........... 59
       B. Alcohol Use and Flying...... 61
       C. Boating Accidents and
          Drownings................... 62
       D. Fires and Burns............. 63
       E. Falls....................... 64
       F. Alcohol Use and Head
          Injuries.................... 64
       G. Alcohol Use and Spinal
          Cord Injuries............... 68
   II. ALCOHOL, CRIME AND VIOLENCE.... 69
       A. Alcohol and Family Violence. 71
   III. ALCOHOL ABUSE AND THE WORK
        ENVIRONMENT.................... 75
       A. Tardiness and Absenteeism... 77
       B. Accidents and Other
          Consequences................ 78

C. Dealing with Alcohol Abuse
         in the Workplace........... 79

CHAPTER 4
ALCOHOLISM, DRUGS AND TOBACCO.......... 93
   I.   ALCOHOLISM.................... 93
   II. DRUG ABUSE.................... 98
   III. TOBACCO.......................103

CHAPTER 5
ALCOHOL AND NUTRITIONAL DEFICIENCIES....111
   I.   VITAMINS......................112
        A. Lipid or Fat Soluble.......112
        B. Water Soluble..............114
   II. MINERALS......................118
   III. AMINO ACIDS...................122
   IV. GLUCOSE.......................123
   V.   LIPIDS, FATS, AND FATTY ACIDS..124

CHAPTER 6
ALCOHOLISM AND THE FAMILY...............137
   I.   ALCOHOL CHILDREN OF
        ALCOHOLICS....................139
   II. EMOTIONAL EFFECTS OF PARENTAL
        ALCOHOLISM ON OFFSPRING.......141
   III. FAMILY VIOLENCE...............142
   IV. STRESS ASSOCIATED WITH
        PARENTAL ALCOHOLISM...........143

CHAPTER 7
ALCOHOL AND HOMELESSNESS................161

CHAPTER 8
ALCOHOL ASSESSMENT TOOLS................169
   I.   ALCOHOL USE EVALUATIONS.........169
        A. Alcohol Use Questionnaire....169
        B. Psychosocial Evaluation......169
   II. TREATMENT MODALITIES............180
        A. Outpatient Clinics..........180
        B. AA, Al-Anon Self-Help Groups.181
        C. Inpatient Treatment.........181

Introduction

I. ALCOHOL AND DISABILITIES

Approximately 27 million people, or 15 percent of the population in the United States over the age of sixteen years, have a disability according to the 1986 Harris Poll. A disability is defined as any health condition that limits or interferes with normal daily or work related activities.[1] The Americans With Disabilities Act of 1990 (ADA) states an individual with a disability is a person who has a physical or mental impairment that substantially limits one or more major life activities, has a record of such a disability, and is regarded by others as having such an impairment. Examples of physical or mental impairments include but are not limited to the following contagious and noncontagious diseases: cancer, cerebral palsy, heart disease, orthopedic, visual, speech, hearing problems, diabetes, HIV/AIDS (symptomatic or asymptomatic), mental retardation, multiple sclerosis, psychiatric illness, epilepsy, specific learning disabilities, drug addiction, and **alcoholism**.[2]

In regard to work disability alone, the National Census for Health Statistics' annual National Health Interview Survey (NHIS) reported that 13.4 million or 8.6 percent of the population between the ages of 16 and 64 have a health problem or disability which has prevented or limited the kind or amount of work that can be done.[3]

Alcoholism, widely accepted as a disability, is a health condition that can limit or interfere with one's normal daily or work related endeavors. In the **Handbook of Severe Disabilities** alcoholism is defined as a person's only disability or a disability that can occur with one or more other physical or

2 Introduction

psychiatric impairments.[4] Alcoholism is also considered by the National Council on Alcoholism and Drug Dependence (NCADD) as a primary, chronic, progressive and potentially fatal disease.[5] It is characterized by denial, tolerance, impaired control over drinking, preoccupation with drinking, and continued use despite adverse physical, psychological, or social consequences. Therefore, when looking at the figure of 15 percent of the population in the United States being disabled, one must determine if the primary disability reported is alcoholism. If the primary disability is not alcoholism, and with the high prevalence of alcoholism and alcohol abuse in the United States, (between 15,000,000 and 22,000,000 Americans) the question must then be posed, how has alcoholism contributed to the existing physical or psychiatric disability reported? Quite often, the occurrence of other physical or psychiatric disabilities is due to the deleterious effects of acute or chronic alcohol consumption. However, the secondary disability or complication of alcoholism, such as head trauma or spinal cord injury resulting from drinking and driving, may be the disability that is reported and alcoholism in this instance may be overlooked.

Alcoholism is a major disability that occurs in both genders as well as in all ethnic, socioeconomic, and age groups. It transcends all occupations and can be diagnosed in professionals as well as unskilled labor and unemployed. Alcoholism is a disease that contributes to a diversity of secondary complications with, at times, irreversible or fatal consequences. The disease of alcoholism can create havoc not only with the individual's physical and psychological well-being, but also contribute to familial and societal dysfunction. Consequently, when looking at broad statistics pertaining to disabilities, it is imperative to determine whether alcoholism is the only disability an individual may be diagnosed with or whether alcoholism is the contributing factor to a myriad of physical and/or mental disabilities.

Although alcoholism falls into the broad definition of types of disabilities, alcoholism is generally not regarded as the primary disability when physical or mental impairments, as a result of alcohol misuse, have surfaced. All too often it is the secondary complication or symptom of alcoholism that receives attention and treatment. For example, in a study of emergency room trauma cases, Roizen concluded that 20 to 37 percent of these cases were a consequence of alcohol abuse or dependence.[6] Another study of 2,262 trauma patients revealed that 93 percent had a blood alcohol determination.[7]

In a random examination of emergency room records pertaining to emergency psychiatric services in a major central New York hospital, alcohol involvement as a primary diagnosis was listed in the minority of cases as compared to the primary psychiatric diagnoses of depression, psychosis or anxiety. However, upon closer scrutiny of incident rates of psychiatric services, alcohol involvement was a hidden rate not accounted for as a primary diagnosis. For example, for the month of December 1987, there were 44.6 percent psychiatric diagnoses and 7.2 percent alcohol diagnoses. However, when records were examined more closely to determine if alcohol was present in any of primary psychiatric diagnoses, alcohol involvement appeared in 32 out of 162 psychiatric contacts. According to these records, alcohol may have contributed to the primary diagnosis of depression or anxiety, yet the psychiatric disorder was listed as the primary diagnosis. If alcohol had been listed as the primary diagnosis which may have contributed to the psychiatric disorder, the number of alcohol incidents for the month of December would have been 19.2 percent instead of 7.2 percent. This same hidden incident rate of alcohol was apparent in three other months chosen at random.[8]

But why the reluctance or hesitance in listing alcohol abuse or dependence as a primary diagnosis? Medical practitioners, unfortunately, tend to overlook the use and abuse of alcohol or other drugs and focus on the physical or psychiatric disorder as the primary diagnosis.[9-12] Failure to diagnose alcoholism may be due to the lack of specialized training in substance abuse disorders. Surveys have revealed that although undergraduate and residency training programs may include instruction in alcohol and drug abuse issues, this instruction unfortunately consists of separate lectures or courses not directly tied to the medical training programs.[13] In the end, and all too often, what ensues is the treatment of the signs and symptoms of the underlying cause of certain physical or psychiatric disorders; namely, alcoholism.

In a review of literature pertaining to head and spinal cord traumas, Houk and Thacker reported that head injuries alone affect 1.3 million people and more than 50,000 individuals survive with severe and chronic disabilities.[14] In addition, between 10,000 and 20,000 individuals suffer from spinal cord injuries annually. In the United States today, there are between 110,000 and 230,000 individuals disabled with serious spinal cord trauma. The national medical costs of treating head and spinal cord injuries are an estimated $9 to $12.5 billion and $4 billion respectively.[15,16] Furthermore, lost earnings as a result of spinal cord injuries alone amount to approximately $3.4 billion per year.[17] The causes of these head and spinal cord injuries were listed as motor vehicle crashes, falls, assaults, and recreational accidents. However, how many of these causes involved alcohol use and abuse? How often does alcohol contribute to the devastating impact of physical and/or mental disabilities? The answer is, all too often. This contiguous occurrence of alcohol misuse and either acute or chronic physical, mental and social consequences will be addressed throughout this text. Except where specifically delineated, the terms alcoholism alcohol abuse and alcohol misuse are used interchangeably.

II. PREVALENCE OF ALCOHOL ABUSE AND DEPENDENCE

Grant and colleagues presented the following data pertaining to the prevalence of alcohol abuse and alcohol dependence in the United States as defined in the **Diagnostic and Statistical Manual of Mental Disorders,** Third Edition, Revised (**DSM-III-R**).[18,19] A nationwide household interview survey was conducted by the National Center for Health Statistics and sponsored by the National Institute on Alcohol Abuse and Alcoholism (NIAAA) with 43,809 individuals aged 18 years and older. All fifty states and the District of Columbia were included in this survey which demonstrated an 85.5 percent response rate. According to the criteria set down by this survey, an individual who exhibited a maladaptive pattern of alcohol use despite adverse social, physical, psychological or vocational consequences was diagnosed with alcohol abuse. Alcohol dependence was diagnosed in an individual when he/she met at least three of the following criteria as defined by the **DSM-III-R**.[20]

1. Alcohol taken in larger amounts or over a longer period than intended.
2. Persistent or one or more unsuccessful efforts to cut down or control alcohol intake.

3. Great deal of time spent in activities to get alcohol, consume alcohol, or recover from its effects.
4. Frequent intoxication or withdrawal symptoms which interfered with ability to fulfill major obligations at work, school, or home.
5. Social, occupational, or recreational activities given up or reduced because of alcohol use.
6. Continued alcohol use despite adverse social, psychological, or physical problems caused by or exacerbated by alcohol use.
7. Marked tolerance and need for increased amounts of alcohol in order to achieve intoxication or desired effect.
8. Withdrawal symptoms.
9. Alcohol consumption to relieve or avoid withdrawal symptoms.

According to the results of this survey, individuals who met the criteria for alcohol abuse, did not meet the criteria for alcohol dependence. The two groups, therefore, were mutually exclusive. Findings of the survey revealed that nearly 9.0 percent adults surveyed (representing 15,295,000 Americans) met **DSM-III-R** criteria for one-year alcohol abuse and dependence. Furthermore, males were three times more likely than females to be diagnosed with either alcohol abuse or dependence. The authors of this survey did not find any differences in the prevalence estimates of alcohol abuse and dependence for the year 1984 which revealed an 8.58 percent prevalence rate for the sample with a corresponding population estimate of 15,100,000 Americans.

In a projection of demographic trends for the period 1985-1995, Williams and colleagues have alleged that if alcohol abuse and alcoholism remain at their present levels, alcohol abuse and alcoholism will have risen an estimated 4 percent. Furthermore, "the number of alcoholics will increase from 10.5

million to 11.2 million (a 7 percent increase), and the number of alcohol abusers will remain stable at 7.2 million."[21] Williams and colleagues have estimated these projections on known demographic changes that will occur in the United States population over the 1985-1995 period, including the rates of alcoholism and alcohol abuse expected in males and females of varying ages. And with the increase of alcoholism and alcohol misuse comes physical, psychological, social and economic consequences.

In 1986, the federal government launched the "war on drugs" campaign. Alcohol was excluded from this strategy. Yet alcohol is responsible for 100,000 deaths annually, strikes one in four American families, and approximately 76 million or 40 percent of Americans live or have lived in alcoholic families.[22] Moreover, according to current statistics, approximately 22 million individuals in the United States is alcoholic and/or suffers the complications of alcohol misuse.[23] This current figure of 22 million Americans who are alcoholics or alcohol abusers is already a greater number then the projected figure of 18.4 million cited earlier by Williams and colleagues. The fact that the current prevalence rate of alcoholism exceeds the projected figures, emphasizes the need to take a serious look at the acute and chronic consequences of alcohol misuse that lead to physical and/or psychiatric disabilities.

III. PREVENTION OF DISABILITIES THROUGH THE PREVENTION OF ALCOHOL MISUSE

Recently prevention research has begun to focus on alcohol abuse and alcohol-related problems. However, prevention efforts must do more than just limit the amount of alcohol an individual consumes. Prevention efforts must take into account several parameters. These

8 Introduction

parameters are short-term and long term consequences of alcohol use, alcohol abuse, and alcohol dependence, including individual, social, and economic consequences. In addition, and of utmost importance, prevention activities pertaining to reduction of developmental disabilities, head and spinal cord injuries, consequences of accidents, crime, and violence, etc. must look into alcohol abuse as a contributing factor to the high incidence and prevalence of these and other disabilities. As Ashley stated, "because alcohol abuse can affect individuals, families, and populations, a broad view of the 'problem of alcohol consumption' is necessary to assess the full range of the effects of alcohol use in society."[24] Alcoholism is a disability that requires in depth attention and investigation into its connection with the myriad of physical and mental disabilities that impair an individual's ability to function to his/her fullest capacity and achieve his/her fullest potential.

In a statement on prevention of human disabilities and recommended policies and practices for the 1980s presented at the fifth Mary E. Switzer Memorial Seminar, Marge outlined 15 primary causes of disabilities.[25] These causes are as follows:
1. Genetic Disorders
2. Perinatal Complications
3. Acute and Chronic Illness
4. Accidents
5. Violence
6. Environmental Problems
7. Alcohol and Drug Abuse
8. Tobacco
9. Nutritional Disorders
10. Educational Deficiency
11. Deleterious Child Rearing Practices
12. Familial Deleterious Beliefs
13. Unsanitary Living Conditions
14. Inaccessibility to Health Care
15. Stress

Although alcohol abuse is listed as one of the primary causes of human disabilities, upon closer investigation it is obvious that alcohol abuse also impacts and contributes to all remaining causes of disabilities. How alcoholism contributes to the causes of preventable disabilities is addressed throughout this text in the following manner.

Chapter 1, **"Alcohol and Fetal Complications,"** addresses genetic disorders and perinatal complications (primary causes of disabilities #1 and #2) that have resulted due to maternal and paternal alcohol consumption. Fetal Alcohol Syndrome (FAS), the leading cause of mental retardation in the United States, and Fetal Alcohol Effects (FAE) are examined in detail. This chapter emphasizes the teratogenic effects of alcohol ingestion on the developing fetus or nursing infant which range from physical complications, behavioral problems, to intellectual impairments.

Chapter 2, **"Alcohol and Acute and Chronic Illness,"** addresses primary causes of disabilities #3 (acute and chronic illness) and #10 (educational deficiency) and presents documentation pertaining to acute and chronic consequences of alcohol consumption. Among the physical and psychiatric impairments discussed are: cancers of the mouth, tongue, pharynx, larynx, esophagitis, gastritis, Mallory-Weiss Syndrome, rectal cancer, pancreatitis, cirrhosis of the liver and other liver ailments, heart disease, cardiomyopathy, hypertension, stroke, pneumococcal pneumonia, sexual dysfunction, breast cancer, educational deficiencies, Korsakoff's Syndrome, Alzheimer's Disease, and alcohol and AIDS.

Chapter 3, **"Alcohol and Adverse Social Consequences,"** addresses primary causes of disabilities #4 (accidents), #5 (violence), and #6 (environmental problems). This chapter is divided into the main categories of Accidents, Crimes and Violence, and Alcohol and the Work Environment. Information is presented as to how alcohol abuse has contributed to the high incidence and prevalence of domestic violence, child abuse, homicides, motor vehicle crashes, and accidents leading to head and spinal cord injuries. This chapter also documents the vast economic consequences resulting from alcohol involvement in relation to the workplace.

Chapter 4, **"Alcohol, Drugs and Tobacco"**, addresses primary causes of disabilities #7 (alcohol/drug abuse) and #8 (tobacco). This chapter outlines the various definitions of alcoholism, including the disease concept. Substantial information is also presented regarding the synergistic effects of alcohol use in combination with other sedative-hypnotic drugs and tobacco.

Chapter 5, **"Alcohol and Nutritional Deficiencies,"** addresses primary causes of disabilities #9 (nutritional disorders). This chapter discusses the impact of alcohol consumption on the depletion of or impact on various vitamins and minerals necessary for the healthy functioning of the human body.

Chapter 6, **"Alcohol and the Family"**, addresses primary causes of disabilities #11 (deleterious child rearing beliefs), #12 (familial deleterious beliefs, and #15 (stress). This chapter discusses at great length the impact of the alcoholic parent(s) on the child. Information is also given pertaining to post-traumatic stress disorder resulting from the dysfunctional family system.

Chapter 7, **"Alcohol and Homelessness,"** addresses primary causes of disabilities #13 (unsanitary living conditions) and #14 (inaccessibility to health care). Information and statistics are given pertaining to homelessness issues and how alcohol abuse has impacted on this population.

Chapter 8, **"Alcohol Assessment Tools"**, provides the reader with two types of evaluations in assessing an individual's involvement with alcohol. The first evaluation is a self-administered, 16-item Alcohol Use Questionnaire. This simple questionnaire addresses a variety of issues pertaining to alcohol use. The second evaluation is the "Comprehensive Psychosocial Evaluation". This evaluation lists questions pertaining to the individual's personal and family history, and alcohol/drug history. Sample questions are presented to assist the reader in identifying the extent of an individual's alcohol history. Incorporated into this evaluation is a section on job performance. The job performance section is specifically geared to the individual's work productivity and relationships on the job. Again, sample questions are given to assist the reader in assessing the individual's extent of alcohol involvement and its impact on the work environment. This chapter also outlines a number of treatment modalities that may be recommended upon the results of the evaluation.

In conclusion, in an investigation of the history of alcohol and man, it was found that there is no period in history that has not made reference to the production, consumption, or deleterious impact of alcoholic beverages. Alcohol abuse has been recognized as a contributing factor to health problems and societal dysfunction dating back to the Code of Hammurabi of Babylonia, 1700 B.C. Furthermore, the disease concept of alcoholism was first suggested by a Roman jurist named Domitus Ulpinus in approximately A.D. 100.[26] Yet today, the deleterious effects of the legal and widely used drug, alcohol, continue to play havoc with individuals, families, and society in general. It is the intent of this book to provide the reader with the understanding and awareness of the myriad of preventable physical and psychiatric disabilities that are caused through alcohol consumption.

REFERENCES

1. Houk, V. N. and Thacker, S. B., The Centers for Disease Control program to prevent primary and secondary disabilities in the United States, **Public Health Reports, 104**, 226, 1989.
2. ADA: Public accommodations and commercial facilities. (Americans with Disabilities Act of 1990, Part 2). **Paraplegia News, 45**, 21, 1991.
3. Kraus, L. E. Disability and work: 13.4 million people have a work disability, **Worklife, 2**, 37, 1989.
4. Fox, V., Conway, J. P., and Schweigler, J., Alcoholism, in **Handbook of Severe Disabilities**, Clowers, S., Ed., U.S. Government Printing Office, Washington, D.C., 1982, chap. 17.
5. National Council on Alcoholism and Drug Dependence (NCADD), **Definition of Alcoholism**, NCADD, New York, 1990.
6. Roizen, J., **Alcohol and Trauma, in Drinking and Casualties: Accidents, Poisonings and Violence in an International Perspective**, Giesbrecht, R., Gonzales, R., Grant, M., Osterberg, E., Room, R., Rootman, I., and Towle, L., Eds., Routledge, London, 1988.
7. Meyers, H. B., Zepeda, S. G., and Murdock, M. A., Alcohol and trauma: An endemic syndrome, **The Western Journal of Medicine, 153**, 149, 1990.
8. Robertson, J. A. and Plant, M. A., Alcohol, sex and risks of HIV infection, **Drug and Alcohol Dependence, 22**(1), 75, 1988.
9. Abbott, J. A., Goldberg, G. A., and Becker, E. B., The role of a medical audit in assessing management of alcoholics with acute pancreatitis, **Quarterly Journal of Studies of Alcohol, 35**, 272, 1974.
10. Cotter, F. and Callahan, C., Training primary care physicians to identify and treat substance abuse, **Alcohol Health and Research World, 11(4)**, 70, 1987.

11. Galanter, M. and Sperber, J., General hospitals in the alcoholism treatment system, in **Encyclopedic Handbook of Alcoholism**, Pattison, E. M. and Kaufman, E., Eds., Gardner Press, New York, pp. 828-836, 1982.

12. Moore, R. A., The prevalence of alcoholism in a community general hospital, **American Journal of Psychiatry, 128**(5), 638, 1971.

13. Cotter, **Training**, 1987.

14. Houk, **Centers**, 1989.

15. Ergas, Z., Spinal cord injury in the United States: A statistical update, **Central Nervous System Trauma, 2**, 19, 1985.

16. Graybow, J. D., Oxford, K. P., and Rieder, M. E., The cost of head trauma in Olmstead County, Minnesota, 1970-1974, **American Journal of Public Health, 74**, 710, 1984.

17. Houk, **Centers**, 1989.

18. Grant, B. F., Harford, T. C., Chou, P., Pickering, R., Dawson, D. A., Stinson, F. S., and Noble, J., Prevalence of DSM-III-R alcohol abuse and dependence: United States 1988, **Alcohol Health and Research World, 15**(1), 9196, 1991.

19. American Psychiatric Association (APA), **Diagnostic and Statistical Manual**, 3rd Ed., revised, American Psychiatric Press, Washington, D. C., 1987.

20. APA, **DSM-III-R**, 1987.

21. Williams, G. D., Stinson, F. S., Parker, D. A., Harford, T. C., and Noble, J., Demographic trends, alcohol abuse and alcoholism: 1985-1995, **Alcohol Health and Research World, 11**(3), 80, 1987.

22. National Council on Alcoholism and Drug Dependence (NCADD), **The War on Drugs: Failure and Fantasy**, NCADD, New York, 1992.

23. Department of Health and Human Services (DHHS), Seventh Special Report to the44 U. S. Congress on Alcohol and Health, **DHHS #RPO757, USDHHS**, Rockville, Maryland, 1990.

24. Ashley, M. J., How extensive is the problem of alcoholism? **Alcohol Health and Research World, 13,** 305, 1989.

25. Marge, M., The prevention of human disabilities: Policies and practices for the 80s, in **International Aspects of Rehabilitation of Disabled Persons: Policy Guidance for the 1980s**, Perlman, L. G., Ed., National Rehabilitation Association, Alexandria, Virginia, pp. 11-22, 1980.

26. O'Brien, R. and Chafetz, M., **The Encyclopedia of Alcoholism**, 2nd Ed., Facts on File, New York, 1991.

Chapter 1

ALCOHOL AND FETAL COMPLICATIONS

I. BIRTH DEFECTS

It is well established that beverage alcohol or ethanol produces defects in offspring in utero. The teratogenic[1] effects on the developing fetus as a result of alcohol ingestion on the part of the pregnant woman range from growth deficiency, to physical malformations, behavioral problems, brain abnormalities to death.[1-3] The reason for this continuum of deleterious effects on the child is the fact that alcohol freely passes through the placental barrier and enters the circulatory system of the developing fetus. Upon ingestion of alcohol, the blood alcohol levels of the fetus are similar to those of the pregnant woman consuming alcohol. Alcohol also crosses the blood-brain barrier and can effect DNA formation, as well as contribute to structural brain abnormalities.[4-6]

Evidence that excessive consumption of alcohol during pregnancy constitutes a hazard to the unborn child dates as far back as 1834. In a report to British Parliament the statement was made that children born to alcoholic mothers had a "starved, shriveled, and imperfect look."[7] Researchers Sullivan, Rouquette, Lemoine and colleagues reported that increased rates of stillbirth, growth retardation, and physical abnormalities existed in offspring of alcoholic women.[8-11]. In 1973 the term "fetal alcohol syndrome" (FAS) was introduced by Jones and Smith to describe a pattern of abnormalities noticed in offspring of alcohol abusing mothers.

---

[1] **Teratogenecity** of alcohol refers to alcohol's ability in producing malformations or deformities.

16 ALCOHOL AND FETAL COMPLICATIONS

Fetal Alcohol Syndrome (FAS), which is a preventable tragedy, is the leading cause of mental retardation in the United States today.[12] FAS presents a recognizable pattern of physical and behavioral abnormalities that is caused by the use of alcohol during the growth of the fetus. The clinical features of FAS are as follows: (1) prenatal and/or postnatal growth retardation, (2) central nervous system (CNS) involvement (signs of neurologic abnormality, developmental delay or intellectual impairment), (3) characteristic facial dysmorphology[13] and (4) major organ system malformations[14].

Effects of alcohol use on behavioral development have been described as follows: (1) disturbed sleep or decreased sleep [15], (2) hyperactivity, decreased attention span, restlessness,[16] (3) problem solving difficulties, impulsivity, speech, and hearing loss or impairment,[17-19]] and (4) mental retardation.[20]

Visual system anomalies are also common in children exposed to alcohol in utero.[21] Strabismus or esotropia (crossed eyes), optic nerve hypoplasia or the reduction in the number of optic nerve axons, and abnormal vasculature (arrangement of blood vessels) in the retina have also been observed.[22]

The Fifth Special Report on Alcohol and Health presented in 1983, noted that "maternal alcohol abuse is the most frequent known environmental cause of mental retardation in the Western World."[23] Alcohol-related mental handicaps and mental retardation are considered to be the most serious of all alcohol related birth defects and the number one preventable birth defect.[24-26] In addition,

> Experts estimate that for every one child diagnosed with FAS, at least 10 others have more subtle and often unrecognized alcohol-caused problems. . . prenatal alcohol exposure may turn

out to be the primary cause of learning disabilities and hyperactivity.[27]

Clarren reported that FAS occurs in 30 to 45 percent of infants born to chronic, heavy daily drinkers.[28] Approximately 40,000 infants are born each year with birth defects as a result of alcohol consumption during pregnancy.[29] Overall, the incidence of FAS has been estimated to occur from 1 to 2.2 to 3 in every 1,000 live births.[30-32] In general, there is a 10 percent chance of giving birth to a child with FAS and a 30 to 40 percent chance of giving birth to a child with Fetal Alcohol Effects (FAE) when the woman is a chronic alcohol drinker.[33] The use of the term "suspected fetal alcohol effects" (FAE) is recommended when only some of the criteria for FAS are apparent.[34]

Researchers (as cited in this section) have determined that alcohol consumption causes damage to the fetus throughout the pregnancy. Numerous animal studies confirm that acetaldehyde, the primary metabolite of alcohol, and alcohol are directly toxic to the developing fetus.[35] Alcohol use negatively affects the developing fetus by collapsing blood vessels, depriving the growing fetus of glucose and oxygen, drying out cells and damaging neurons and the developing brain.[36] Alcohol consumption during the first trimester has been linked with morphologic abnormalities such as low nasal bridge, thin upper lip, and microcephaly. Consumption of alcohol during the second trimester carries with it a greater risk of miscarriage. Third trimester alcohol drinking results in decreased fetal growth and congenital anomalies.[37,38]

Day and colleagues noted that alcohol consumption during the second and third trimester was connected with a decrease in infant body length; five and ten millimeters respectively. Day and colleagues also estimated that for every alcoholic drink per day during the third trimester, there was a decrease of five millimeters in infant head circumference.[39] In addition to infant size, heavy use of alcohol during pregnancy was shown to affect fetal heart development.[40]

In addition to the damage alcohol consumption can do to the developing fetus, Lele noted that heavy drinking at least one month prior to conception also produced complications since the embryo is susceptible to the effects of alcohol prior to and after conception.[41]

Intellectual impairments on the part of the child exposed to alcohol in utero are especially disturbing in that FAS or FAE often go undiagnosed and affected children are not given adequate follow-up care.[42] Whereas full FAS symptoms appear only when a woman has been drinking alcohol excessively throughout her pregnancy, experts estimate that three to four times as many children are born with FAE.[43] Full FAS may be easier to detect and diagnose due to facial and physical abnormalities of the newborn, however, FAE is very difficult to diagnose at birth.[44] Often FAE is not detected until the child goes to school and even then in utero exposure to alcohol may not be acknowledged as the cause of many of the learning problems the child experiences. Marino and colleagues have acknowledged that FAE has a long latent period before it is diagnosed correctly.[45]

However, it is not surprising that FAE may go undiagnosed. In a recent study conducted by Little and colleagues, one of the largest neonatal units in the United States failed to diagnose FAS in infants whose mothers had a documented history of alcohol abuse during pregnancy and the infants had physical features consistent with FAS as described in the medical records. The hospital staff had a 100% failure rate of diagnosing FAS in this research study's sample. Little and colleagues concluded that there appears to be an underestimate of the prevalence of FAS and even more likely an underestimate of infants with FAE.[46]

Children with FAE exhibit lower IQs, poor memory skills, short attention spans, impulsivity and poor judgment. Furthermore, children with "mild cases of FAE fail to learn from experience either in a skill like learning multiplication tables and telling time, or in a behavior situation. They continue to repeat behaviors that they have been warned about in the past."[47] Approximately 33,000 children who show intellectual impairments and general school failure are victims of FAE.[48] It is apparent from these research studies that fetal alcohol exposure may be the contributing factor to learning disorders.

It is important to note, that African-American women who abuse alcohol during pregnancy are at a seven times greater risk of exposing their unborn children to FAS.[49] However, the reason for this higher risk is unknown at this time.[50] Researchers have identified that whereas abstention is more common among African-American men, African-American women who drink are more likely than white women to drink heavily.[51]

Are drinking fathers endangering their unborn children? Researchers at the Washington University of Medicine in St. Louis put 15 male rats on a diet similar to an adult alcoholic for one month. The rats were taken off the alcohol two weeks before breeding. At first the offspring seemed normal. However, before the rats reached maturity, they began to exhibit signs of learning difficulties. It appeared that the offspring of "alcoholic rats" took 50 percent more time in learning new tasks as compared with rats with non-alcoholic fathers.[52] It is difficult to generalize from an animal sample to the human population, however, this research nonetheless poses some very important questions. Although no evidence based on human samples exists of paternal alcohol use and pregnancy, fertilization with defective sperm (due to prolonged use of alcohol by the father) may result in fetal anomalies.[53]

II. PERINATAL COMPLICATIONS

Perinatal refers to the period beginning after the 28th week of pregnancy through 28 days following birth. Overall, the effects of alcohol abuse during pregnancy and delivery are as follows: vaginal bleeding experienced by the alcoholic mother, premature separation of the placenta, and fetal distress.[54]

Low birth weight and intrauterine growth retardation is associated with significant increases in risk for fetal and infant mortalities and long-term abnormalities in neurologic development and intelligence. Sokol and Little provide evidence linking in utero alcohol exposure and decreased fetal growth.[55,56] Diminished prenatal growth is dose related and is more severe in the third trimester or after the 28th week of pregnancy.[57,58] Day and colleagues reported that alcohol-exposed infants were not only smaller at birth but also had a decreased rate of growth during their first six to eight months.[59] In a review of literature, Bjerre & Hansen wrote that low birthweight (LBW) predisposes the infant to lesions of the CNS with impairment of intellect and behavior disorders. In their study of 144 LBW children (less then 2500 g) aged seven years, Bjerre and Hansen found that on the average the intellectual level of the LBW children was lower than the comparison group. The Bjerre and Hansen study also confirmed earlier findings that LBW children had more problems in school then children in general.[60]

Other studies have revealed that during an eight-month study of infants exposed to alcohol before birth, difficulty in feeding was noted and a positive relationship was found between maternal alcohol consumption and infant feeding problems.[61] There is also a significant correlation between maternal alcohol use, smoking and low birthweight. Offspring of mothers who both drank heavily and smoked during pregnancy delivered babies that weighed 500 grams less than babies of non-drinking, non-smoking mothers. The synergistic effect of drinking and smoking is an important factor in infant mortality and impaired mental and physical development.[62]

The adverse effects of alcohol use on infant behavioral development may be divided into four main categories: sleep problems in the newborn, hyperactivity, mental retardation, and learning disabilities.[63,64] Maternal use of alcohol during pregnancy is related to decreased attention span and a longer reaction time. It is obvious that alcohol use by pregnant women can have long term behavioral effects in children.[65,66] Several studies have attested to the permanence of functional deficits, behavioral abnormalities, and attention deficits on offspring of alcoholic mothers.[67-69]

The mother ingesting alcohol during pregnancy is not the only risk to the child. Researchers report that there is a positive relationship between maternal alcohol consumption and breast feeding and deleterious effects on the motor development of the newborn. In fact it was found that the greater the amount of alcohol the nursing mother consumed the greater the negative effect on the child.[70] Little and colleagues concluded that the development of muscle control was significantly lowered in infants exposed to alcohol ingested through breast milk.[71] Hudnall reported that alcohol secreted in breast milk has a negative effect on the brain cells of the child until the age of two

22 ALCOHOL AND FETAL COMPLICATIONS

years.[72] Nursing infants of alcohol consuming mothers appear more irritable, drowsy and have abnormal weight gain.[73]

Often it has been the practice of many maternity hospitals and practitioners to encourage drinking wine or beer in helping the process of breast-feeding. However, the deleterious effects of consuming alcohol on the unborn child or the newborn either while pregnant or when breastfeeding far outweigh any possible benefits of having a glass of wine, beer, etc. for relaxation.

SUMMARY

The teratogenic actions of alcohol are well substantiated. In utero exposure to alcohol exists on a continuum "ranging from gross morphological defects at one extreme to more subtle cognitive-behavioral dysfunctions at the less severe end."[74] It is irrefutable that alcohol ingestion during pregnancy causes FAS and FAE. Furthermore, alcohol consumption during breastfeeding has a negative impact on the normal cognitive and behavioral development of the child.

Today, the U. S. Surgeon General, the American Medical Association and the March of Dimes Birth Defects Foundation all agree that there is no known "safe" level of drinking alcohol.[75] Former Surgeon General, C. Everett Koop stated:

> "Even without all the answers, there are two things that are beyond dispute. First, the more the mother drinks, the greater are the risks she takes with the health of her unborn baby. Second, there is no possibility of having a baby with any alcohol-related birth defects - including FAS - if the mother does not drink at all. . . The safest and wisest choice is to avoid alcohol."[76]

Since there are many definitions of what constitutes a light drinker, a moderate drinker, or a heavy drinker, and how much alcohol might effect the child, the best rule of thumb for the parent is "don't drink."

REFERENCES

1. Clarren, S. K., Alvord, E. C., Jr., Sumi, S. M., Streissguth, A. P., and Smith, D. W., Brain malformations related to prenatal exposure to ethanol, **Journal of Pediatrics, 92**(1), 64, 1978.
2. Streissguth, A. P., Barr, H. M., and Martin, D. C., Maternal alcohol use and neonatal habituation assessed with the **Brazelton Scale, Child Development, 54**, 1109, 1983.
3. Streissguth, A. P., Clarren, S. K., and Jones, K. L., A natural history of the fetal alcohol syndrome: A 10-year followup of 11 patients, **Alcohol Health and Research World, 10**(1), 13, 1985.
4. Brown, N. A., Goulding, E. H., and Fabro, S., Ethanol embryotoxicity: Direct effects on mammalian embryos in vitro, **Science, 206**, 573, 1979.
5. Clarren, **Brain**, 1978.
6. Radcliffe, A., Rush, P., Sites, C. F., and Cruse, J., **Pharmer's Almanac: Pharmacology of Drugs**, MAC Publishing, Denver, Colorado, 1989.
7. Ray, O. and Ksir, C., **Drugs, Society and Human Behavior**, Times Mirror/Mosby, St. Louis, Missouri, 1987.
8. Sullivan, W. C., A note on the influence of maternal inebriety on the offspring, **Journal Mental Science, 45**, 489-503, 1899.
9. Rouquette, J., **Influence of Parental Alcoholic Toxicomania on the Physical and Psychic Development of Young Children**, Unpublished doctoral dissertation in medicine, University of Paris.

10. Lemoine, P., Harrouseau, H., and Borteyru, J. P., Les enfants de parents alcooliques: Anomalies observees, **Quest Medicine, 25**, 476-482.

11. Clarren, S. K., Recognition of fetal alcohol syndrome, **Journal of the American Medical Association, 245**(23), 2436-2439, 1981.

12. Streissguth, A. P., Aase, J. M., Clarren, S. K., Randels, S. P., LaDue, R. A., and Smith, D. F., Fetal alcohol syndrome in adolescents and adults, **The Journal of the American Medical Association, 265**, 1961-1967, 1991.

13. Lele, A. S., Fetal alcohol syndrome, **New York State Journal of Medicine, 82**(8), July, 1982.

14. Clarren, **Recognition**, 1981.

15. Rosett, H. L., Snyder, P., Sander, L. W., Lee, A., Cook, P., Weiner, L., and Gould, J., Effects of maternal drinking on neonate state regulation, **Developmental Medicine and Child Neurology, 21**, 464-473, 1979.

16. Shaywitz, S. E., Cohen, D. J. and Shaywitz, B. A., Behavior and learning difficulties in children of normal intelligence born to alcoholic mothers, **Journal of Pediatrics, 96**, 978-982, 1980.

17. Church, M. W. and Gerkin, K. P. Hearing disorders in children with fetal alcohol syndrome: Findings from case reports, **Pediatrics, 82**(2), 147-154, 1988.

18. Streissguth, A. P. and LaDue, R. A., Psychological and behavioral effects in children prenatally exposed to alcohol, **Alcohol Health and Research World, 10**(1), 6-12, 1985.

19. Streissguth, A. P. Sampson, P. D., and Barr, H. M., Neurobehavioral dose-response effects of prenatal alcohol exposure in humans from infancy to adulthood, **Annals of the New York Academy of Sciences, 562**, 145-158, 1989.

20. Abel, E. L., Behavioral teratology of alcoholic beverages compared to ethanol, **Neurobehavioral Toxicology and Teratology, 3**, 339-342, 1981.

21. Department of Health and Human Services (DHHS), **Seventh Special Report to the U.S. Congress on Alcohol and Health**, DHHS Rep. #RP0757, USDHHS, Rockville, Maryland, January 1990.

22. Stromland, K., Ocular involvement in the fetal alcohol syndrome, **Surv Ophthalmology, 31**, 277-284, 1987.

23. Ray, **Drugs**, 1987.

24. Abel, **Fetal**, 1986.

25. Dorris, M., Fetal alcohol syndrome, **Parents' Magazine, 65**, 238-242.

26. Streissguth, **Neurobehavioral**, 1989.

27. Brody, J. E., Fetal alcohol syndrome: Evidence mounts that babies and booze don't mix, **New York Times News Service, Syracuse Herald Journal**, AA2, January 26, 1986.

28. Clarren, **Recognition**, 1981.

29. Newman, L. F. and Papkalla, U. K., Many causes of learning disorders are avoidable, **Brown University Child Behavior and Development Letter, 5**, 1-4, 1989.

30. Little, B. B., Snell, L. H., Rosenfeld, C. R., Gilstrap, L. C. III, and Gant, N. F., Failure to recognize fetal alcohol syndrome in newborn infants, **American Journal of Diseases of Children, 144**, 1142-1146, 1990.

31. Nace, E. P., **The Treatment of Alcoholism**, Brunner/Mazel, New York, 1987.

32. Newman, **Many causes**, 1989.

33. Dorris, **Fetal**, 1990.

34. Clarren, S. K., Alvord, E. C. Jr., Sumi, S. M., Streissguth, A. P., and Smith, D. W., Brain malformations related to prenatal exposure to ethanol, **The Journal of Pediatrics, 92**(1), 64-67, 1978.

35. Cook, P. S., Peterson, R. C., and Moore, D. T., **Alcohol, Tobacco, and Other Drugs May Harm the Unborn**, U. S. Department

of Health and Human Services, Rockville, Maryland, 1990.

36. Hudnall, M., Alcohol poses many health risks, few benefits, **Environmental Nutrition, 12**(2), 1, 1989.

37. Rosett, **Effects**, 1979.

38. Rosett, H. L., Weiner, L., Zuckerman, B., McKinley, S., and Edelin, K., Reduction of alcohol consumption during pregnancy with benefits to newborn, **Alcohol: Clinical and Experimental Research, 4**, 178-184, 1980.

39. Day, N. L., Richardson, G., Robles, N., Sambamoorthi, U., Taylor, P., Scher, M., Stoffer, D., Jasperse, D., and Cornelius, M., Effect of prenatal alcohol exposure on growth and morphology of offspring at eight months of age, **Pediatrics, 85**, 748-752, 1990.

40. Davidson, D. M., Cardiovascular effects of alcohol, **Western Journal of Medicine, 151**, 430-440, 1989.

41. Lele, **Fetal**, 1982.

42. Little, **Failure**, 1990.

43. Dorris, **Fetal**, 190.

44. Havey, E. A., Fetal alcohol syndrome, **Pediatrics for Parents**, 6-7, July/August 1991.

45. Marino, R. V., Scholl, T. O., Karp, R. J., Yanoff, J. M., and Hetherington, J., Minor physical anomalies and learning disability: What is the prenatal component? **Journal of the National Medical Association, 79(1)**, 37-39.

46. Little, **Failure**, 1990.

47. Havey, **Fetal**, 1991.

48. Newman, **Many causes**, 1989.

49. Sokol, R. J., Ager, J., Martier, S., Debanne, S., Ernhart, C., Kuzma, J., and Miller, S. I., Significant determinants of susceptibility to alcohol teratogenicity, **Annals of New York Academy of Sciences, 477**, 87-102, 1986.

50. National Institute on Alcohol Abuse and Alcoholism, Fetal alcohol syndrome, **Alcohol Alert**, #13.PH297, NIAAA, Rockville Maryland, July 1991.

51. Bradley, A. M., A capsule review of the state of the art: The sixth special report to the U. S. Congress on alcohol and health, **Alcohol Health and Research World, 11**(4), 4-9, 1987.

52. Edell, D., Drinking and fatherhood may not mix, Washington University of Medicine in St. Louis research, **Edell Health Letter, 9**, 6, April 1990.

53. Anderson, R. A., Furby, J. E., Oswald, C., and Zaneveld, L. J. D., Teratological evaluation of mouse fetuses after paternal alcohol ingestion, **Neurobehavioral Toxicology and Teratology, 3**, 117-120, 1981.

54. Cook, **Alcohol**, 1990.

55. Sokol, R. J., Alcohol-in-pregnancy: Clinical research problems, **Neurobehavioral Toxicology and Teratology, 2**, 157-165, 1980.

56. Little, R. E., Moderate alcohol use during pregnancy and decreased infant birth weight, **American Journal of Public Health, 6**, 1154-1156, 1977.

57. Cook, **Alcohol**, 1990.

58. Lochry, E. A., Randall, C. L., Goldsmith, A. A., and Sutker, P. B., Effects of acute alcohol exposure during selected days of gestation in C3H mice, **Neurobehavioral Toxicology and Teratology, 4**, 15-19, 1982.

59. Day, **Effect**, 1990.

60. Bjerre, I. and Hansen, E., Psychomotor development and school-adjustment of 7-year-old children with low birthweight, **Acta Paediatr Scand, 65**, 88-96, 1976.

61. Day, **Effect**, 1990.

62. Edell, D., Smoking, drinking and nose sprays, **Edell Health Letter, 8**, 5, August 1989.

63. Abel, **Behavioral**, 1981.

64. Kruse, J., Alcohol use during pregnancy, **American Family Physician, 29**(4), 199-203, 1984.

65. Landesman-Dwyer, S., Ragozin, A. S., and Little, R. E., Behavioral correlates of

prenatal alcohol exposure: A four-year follow-up study, **Neurobehavioral Toxicology and Teratology,** **3**, 187-193, 1981.

66. Streissguth, A. P., Barr, H. M., and Martin, D. C., Maternal alcohol use and neonatal habituation assessed with the Brazelton Scale, **Child Development, 54,** 1109-1118, 1983.

67. Abel, E. L. and Dintcheff, B. A., Effects of prenatal alcohol exposure on nose poking in year-old rats, **Alcohol, 3,** 210-214, 1986.

68. Aronson, M., Kyllerman, M., Sabel, K. G., Sandin, B., and Olegard, R., Children of alcoholic mothers: Developmental, perceptual, and behavioral characteristics as compared to matched controls, **Acta Paediatrica Scandanavia, 74,** 27-35, 1985.

69. Spohr, H. L. ad Steinhausen, H. C., Follow-up studies of children with fetal alcohol syndrome. **Neuropediatrics, 18,** 13-17, 1987.

70. Drinking and breast feeding, **Pediatrics for Parents, 7,** January 1990.

71. Little, R. E, Anderson, K. W., Ervin, C. H., Worthington-Roberts, B., and Clarren, S. K., Maternal alcohol use during breast feeding and infant mental and motor development at one year, **New England Journal of Medicine, 321,** 425-431, 1989.

72. Hudnall, **Alcohol,** 1989.

73. Cook, **Alcohol,** 1990.

74. Department of Health and Human Services, **Fifth,** 1983.

75. Havey, **Fetal,** 1991.

76. Association for Retarded Citizens (ARC), **Have You Heard About Alcohol and Pregnancy,** ARC, Arlington, Texas, 1986.

Chapter 2

ALCOHOL AND ACUTE OR CHRONIC ILLNESS

I. ACUTE AND CHRONIC ILLNESS

Alcoholism is one of the most prevalent disabilities in the United States.[1] However, it is a disease or disability that creates additional debilitating factors, or other disabilities, for the individual. It is estimated that approximately one-third of all causes of preventable death in the United State are directly related to alcohol abuse.[2] Gloeckner reported that "dozens of diseases are caused entirely, or in part, by the abuse of alcohol. Some of them are killers."[3]

Since many of the life threatening effects of alcohol abuse are directly linked to the toxic effects of alcohol ingestion, many of the harmful consequences of alcohol abuse may be prevented. Frequently, physical complications are a direct result of prolonged exposure to alcohol. The larger the daily dose of alcohol consumption, the higher the risk of serious disease or illness.[4] The following are the most significant adverse complications of alcohol abuse:

1. Mouth

Cancers of the mouth, tongue, pharynx (back of throat), and larynx (voice box) occur more frequently in alcohol abusing individuals than in nonalcoholics.[5-7] Two contributing factors to this increased risk of cancer are (1) deficiencies in Vitamins A, B and zinc found in alcoholics,[8-9] as well as, (2) a synergistic effect between drinking alcohol and smoking.[10-14] Researchers have found that alcoholics smoke at a higher rate than a comparison population; thus increasing the risk of oral cancer.[15-17] It is also important to note that mouthwash users have a

30   ALCOHOL AND ACUTE OR CHRONIC ILLNESS

higher than average incidence of oral cancers, suggesting that ethanol may be topically carcinogenic since mouthwash is seldom swallowed.[18]

2. Esophagus

Cancer of the esophagus (swallowing tube) has been associated with alcohol abuse.[19-22] In addition, the use of both alcohol and tobacco have been identified as strongly related to increased risk in esophageal cancer.[23-25] Esophagitis, a non-malignant inflammation of the esophagus, has also been associated with long-term alcohol abuse.[26]

3. Stomach and Small Intestine

Chronic alcohol use causes an erosion of the stomach lining. This erosion or inflammation of the mucous membranes lining the stomach is known as gastritis and is the most common result of chronic alcohol use.[27] Twenty-five percent of all acute gastritis cases are found in alcoholics as compared to five percent of acute gastritis episodes in nonalcoholics.[28] It is also one of the most common signs of gastrointestinal disease associated with acute or chronic alcohol abuse and results in blood loss or gastric hemorrhaging caused by an increase of stomach acid which damages the stomach lining.[29-31] The Mallory-Weiss syndrome, which refers to bleeding caused by lacerations of the stomach lining, accounts for 5 to 14 percent of gastrointestinal bleeding incidents in hospitalized individuals of whom 60 to 80 percent reported heavy alcohol intake prior to the episode.[32]

Continued bleeding from the stomach lining may also result in ulcers and is one of the main reasons individuals with ulcers are instructed to abstain from alcohol.[33-34] Left untreated, an ulcer may become a bleeding ulcer and result in death.[35] The duodenum, or the first part of the small intestine, may also be adversely effected by chronic alcohol use resulting in a duodenal ulcer or the creation of small lesions.[36-37]

Since the small intestine is also an important site for the absorption of vitamins, minerals, or proteins into the blood stream, the chronic use of alcohol also impairs the body's ability in effectively using these nutrients. Although alcohol may add a high number of calories, it does not provide the individual with the essential vitamins, minerals, protein or fiber necessary for the healthy functioning of the body. Consequently, malnutrition may be the result of chronic alcohol use.[38-40] (A discussion on nutritional disorders caused by alcohol use may be found in Chapter 5).

Although the National Institute on Alcohol Abuse and Alcoholism (NIAAA) cites no clear evidence concerning the connection between alcohol abuse and stomach cancer, Schuckit reports that chronic alcohol use is associated with stomach cancer as well as cancers of the esophagus, head and neck.[41-42]

4. Colon/Rectum

Researchers from the Kaiser Permanente Medical Center in Oakland, California reported that chronic use of alcohol increased the risk of rectal cancer threefold. Also, heavy alcohol drinkers were twice as likely to develop colorectal cancer as compared with light or nondrinkers.[43] Research conducted in Japan with 26,118 adults aged 40 years and over revealed a striking association between alcohol consumption and cancer of the sigmoid colon in both genders. A higher association was observed between alcohol and colon cancer among daily beer drinkers.[44]

5. Pancreas

The pancreas performs two key roles in the human body; (1) the pancreas assists in the breakdown of digested food, and (2) it regulates blood sugar levels.[45] The pancreas is highly susceptible to injury caused by the chronic use of alcohol.

Approximately 40 percent of all individuals with pancreatitis are considered chronic alcohol dependent.[46] Pancreatitis or the painful inflammation of the pancreas which is characterized by severe abdominal pain, nausea and vomiting, may occur ten to fifteen years after heavy drinking.[47] Severe cases of acute pancreatitis may be fatal. However, chronic pancreatitis may be irreversible, and longstanding.[48] In fact, "progressive destruction of the pancreas continues even after the individual stops drinking."[49]

Pancreatic cancer, the fifth leading cause of death due to cancer in the United States, has also been linked with alcohol abuse. Researchers contend that four or more drinks of alcohol on a daily basis may increase the risk of pancreatic cancer by a factor of 2.7.[50] However, Farrow and Davis contend that the role of alcohol in relation to pancreatic cancer remains inconclusive and requires further study.[51]

6. Alcohol and the Liver

The liver is the largest glandular organ in the body and is involved in filtering blood and secreting bile into the gastrointestinal tract. Rubin reported that because the liver is involved in many of the metabolic functions of the body, damage to the liver can have widespread and serious medical consequences for the individual. Secondary complications due to the liver damage are kidney failure, gastrointestinal bleeding, brain disorders, and changes in blood chemistry.[52]

The liver is the primary site of alcohol metabolism or alcohol detoxification.[53] The liver is also the organ most commonly thought to be affected by chronic alcohol use.[54] In fact, chronic liver disease is the most common medical consequence of alcoholism.[55] Alcohol abuse can produce various liver ailments; e.g., alcoholic fatty liver, alcoholic hepatitis, and cirrhosis of the liver.

Fatty liver refers to the damage caused by the infiltration of fatty cells into the normal liver as a result of excessive alcohol intake.[56] A fatty liver is a benign and reversible condition that is not considered serious.[57-58] However, a fatty liver may also be the first stage of alcoholic liver disease if chronic alcohol intake does not cease.[59]

Alcoholic hepatitis is a more serious condition of chronic alcohol use and considered to be the second stage of alcoholic liver disease. During this stage there is an increased destruction of liver tissue causing various degrees of liver inflammation and impairment.[60-62] Symptoms of alcoholic hepatitis include jaundice, low-grade fever, dark urine and an enlarged and tender liver. Left untreated, death can result from liver failure. If abstinence is followed, nearly 80 percent of all individuals experiencing alcoholic hepatitis will recover. However, if drinking is continued, 50 to 80 percent will develop cirrhosis of the liver.[63] Alcoholic hepatitis can occur without the individual experiencing a fatty liver.[64]

Alcoholic cirrhosis is an advanced stage of liver degeneration and is related to prolonged and high levels of alcohol abuse. Cirrhosis of the liver is considered to be an extreme manifestation of the damage caused by chronic alcohol abuse.[65] Cirrhosis is the seventh leading cause of death in the United States, [66-68] and the leading cause of death in alcoholics.[69] Within the Native American population, cirrhosis of the liver is 4.5 times higher than in the general population.[70]

Cirrhosis of the liver may be characterized by diffuse liver cell damage and the formation of scar-like or non-functional tissue. Scar tissue obstructs the flow of blood and the result is a decreased ability of the liver to function properly.[71] The development of jaundice, as a result of impaired liver functioning, means that toxins are accumulating in the blood. Once jaundice develops in the liver, cancer may also develop.[72] An estimated 30 percent of all individuals with diagnosed severe cirrhosis will contract cancer, as compared to 5 percent of patients with mild or moderate cirrhosis.[73]

The liver of an individual with cirrhosis also has difficulty removing toxins, which may build up in the blood. This toxin accumulation can lead to personality changes and even coma. Signs of toxin buildup in the brain include personal neglect, forgetfulness, difficulty in concentrating, or changes in sleeping habits.[74]

Cirrhosis is not reversible. However, it can be arrested through alcohol abstention. The individual will be able to maintain adequate functioning with mild cirrhosis. Although it is believed that cirrhosis is preceded by alcoholic hepatitis, this has not been established.[75] Researchers also report that chronic alcohol ingestion produces cirrhosis of the liver regardless of the individual's nutritional state. In other words, even individuals that maintain a healthy diet may cause damage to the liver through prolonged use of alcohol.[76]

7. Alcohol and the Heart

Heart disease has been directly linked to alcoholism.[77] Alcohol is considered "cardiotoxic" or specifically toxic to the muscle tissue of the heart.[78] Alcohol use can cause arrhythmias (heart beat irregularities);[79-82] endocarditis or the inflammation of the lining membrane of the heart;[83] cardiac fibrillation;[84] subclinical depression of left ventricular function;[85] and cardiomyopathy or the disease of the heart muscle.[86-88]

Clinicians have found that cardiomyopathy, a primary disorder of the heart muscle, is found in chronic heavy drinkers.[89] Symptoms of alcoholic cardiomyopathy include chronic shortness of breath, chest pain, fatigue, palpitations and blood-stained sputum.[90] Alcoholic cardiomyopathy is also a long-recognized cause of congestive heart failure. However, if the individual abstains from drinking, recovery from cardiomyopathy is good but very slow.[91]

Researchers have reported that alcohol and how it affects the heart size is dose related.[92,93] A linear correlation seems to exist between lifetime consumption of alcohol and increased heart size. Researchers have determined that the cause of the enlarged heart is due to muscle fibers of the heart becoming damaged and the heart attempting to compensate for muscle fiber death or damage by enlarging.[94]

8. Alcohol and Musculoskeletal System

In addition to the deleterious effects on the heart muscle, alcohol consumption is also associated with morphological changes in muscle tissue and muscle weakness.[95,96] Acute alcoholic myopathy, an alcohol-induced disorder, has been associated with alcohol abuse for about 120 years.[97,98] Pain, cramps, and muscular weakness are often associated with "the morning after" an alcoholic binge. In this case, muscles become swollen and bruised indicating a certain degree of muscle tissue death.[99] In some instances, kidney failure may occur due to dead muscle tissue floating through the blood stream and obstructing the kidney.

As with the heart, the damage done to the muscle system is alcohol dose related; the more the alcoholic drinks, the weaker the muscles become.[100] Chronic myopathy is not only painful but may also be fatal. Fortunately, symptoms disappear once the individual abstains from alcohol.[101]

Chronic alcohol use also has toxic effects on bone tissue and can result in reduced bone formation, alcohol-induced osteoporosis, increased incidence of fractures,[102] osteopemia or atrophy of the bone, and non-traumatic idiopathic osteonecrosis of the femoral head characterized hip pain.[103]

9. Alcohol and Blood Disorders

An increase in MCV (mean corpuscular volume or average blood cell size) is the most common blood disorder found in alcohol abusing individuals.[104] An increased MCV means that red blood cells are larger in size than normal. Researchers report that approximately 90% of all alcoholics are found to have an increased MCV.[105,106] A blood test is routinely done to determine alcoholism based on MCV levels.[107,108]

Alcohol abusing individuals may also suffer from anemia which can result from decreased red blood cell formation, riboflavin deficiency or folic acid deficiency.[109,110]

Moderate to heavy drinking can also impede absorption of Vitamin K which can reduce the body's blood-clotting ability.[111] A decrease in platelet function can interfere with the platelets sticking together, thereby allowing the person to bleed more easily. [112]

Continually high levels of alcohol in the blood can change the chemistry of the body and result in hypoglycemia.[113] With hypoglycemia, the individual feels weak and sick due to low blood sugar. With severely abnormal low blood sugar the individual may go into a coma.

Hyperlipidemia is another change in blood chemistry in the heavy drinker. With hyperlipidemia, the individual's blood contains higher levels of lipids or fats than normal.

Left untreated, hyperlipidemia may increase the risk of hardening of the arteries and heart disease.[114]

Chronic alcohol ingestion can also result in decreased white blood cell (WBC) production. The individual then may increase the risk of contracting infections since WBC's are important in the body's defense system.[115]

10. Alcohol, Hypertension and Stroke

Alcohol use is related to blood pressure and hypertension. The prevalence of hypertension appears to be significantly related to high levels of alcohol use.[116-118] Hudnall reported that "excessive alcohol intake may be the most common cause of secondary hypertension (high blood pressure for which the cause is known)."[119] Hypertension is 1.6 to 2.4 times more prevalent in heavy drinkers than in non-drinkers.

Chronic alcohol use has also been strongly correlated with an increased risk for stroke.[120-123] Since hypertension is a risk factor for stroke, researchers suggested that the relationship between high levels of alcohol intake and stroke may be mediated by way of alcohol-induced hypertension.[124,125]

11. Alcohol and Pulmonary Disease

In general, pneumococcal pneumonia is more likely to occur in alcoholics than in non-drinking individuals. Aspirative pneumonia, the process whereby the individual while vomiting aspirates contents from the stomach back into the lungs, is also found in alcoholics.[126,127]

The presence of blisters also known as localized pneumatoceles or bullous formations have been observed in chest x-rays of alcoholics. A diagnosis of bullous changes has been associated with alcohol dependence.[128] It is hypothesized that alcohol abusing individuals develop subclinical destruction of cells in the lung tissue in reaction to chronic ingestion of large amounts of alcohol. This destruction of cells continues until the individual abstains from alcohol. However, permanent and irreversible damage to the lung tissue, has been seen in alcoholics.[129]

12. Alcohol and Endocrine System

Individuals with diabetes are at high risk for developing severe and life-threatening reactions to alcohol ingestion.[130] Chronic alcohol consumption can lead to a buildup of two kinds of acid in the bloodstream resulting in lactic acidosis or ketosis. Hypoglycemia (low blood sugar) may also result and possibly be fatal. In addition, the risk of heart attack and stroke (already high in a diabetic) is increased with the ingestion of alcohol.[131,132]

Researchers contend that alcohol consumption over a long period of time can create physiological changes similar to diabetes in individuals not diagnosed with this disease. The reason for this similarity is due to alcohol inhibiting the secretion of insulin from the pancreas; "less glucose is removed from the blood and more glucose is excreted in the urine."[133]

13. Alcohol and Sexual Dysfunction

Regarding gonadal and adrenal effects, researchers have reported that 70 to 80 percent of alcoholic men were found to have decreased libido or impotence.[134,135] This is due to alcohol decreasing testosterone levels and directly damaging testicular form and function. In fact, pertaining to reproductive functioning, alcohol abuse has either a direct or indirect adverse effect in both men and women. In the male, endocrine abnormalities can seriously affect the reproductive functioning due to reduced sperm production, testicular atrophy and loss of secondary characteristics.[136,137] In the female, decreased fertility, infrequent menstrual cycles and amenorrhea have been reported due to chronic alcohol ingestion.[138-140]

In addition to impaired reproductive functioning, chronic alcohol ingestion results in the male producing excessive estrogen (female hormone), and thereby experiencing enlarged mammary glands and feminine pubic hair patterns.[141] In contrast, the female alcoholic shows severe gonadal failure commonly manifested as loss of secondary sex characteristics such as breast and pelvic fat accumulation.[142]

14. Alcohol and Breast Cancer

The National Cancer Institute indicated that 9 percent, or 1 in every 11 women in the United States, will develop breast cancer.[143] Breast cancer is still the most common cancer to strike women. Researchers in the last 20 years have concluded that a strong link exists between alcohol consumption and breast cancer.[144-146] Clinicians contend that there is a 30 percent increase in the risk for breast cancer with moderate alcohol consumption and as much as 50 percent with heavy alcohol use.[147] Case controlled studies have suggested that women who drink are 1.5 to 2 times more likely to develop breast cancer than women who do not consume alcohol.[148] Since breast cancer is one of the largest single causes of female cancer deaths in the United States, and a positive association has been identified between alcohol consumption and breast cancer, it is wise for women to seriously consider the risks associated with drinking alcohol.

15. Alcohol and the Brain

The deleterious effects of alcohol on the brain can be divided into three categories; short-term use/low to moderate doses, short-term use/high doses and long-term use. Short-term use/low to moderate dose effects are those that appear quickly after one drink of alcohol and usually disappear within a few hours after the person stops drinking. Short-term use/low to moderate dose effects include depression of the inhibitory and behavioral control centers of the brain, impaired memory, concentration difficulties, perceptual distortions and decreased insight, attention and reaction time.[149-152]

As the level of drinking increases, normal cognitive functioning decreases. Short-term use/high dose effects include perceptual and motor dysfunctions, and greatly impaired judgment and memory functions. Memory impairment may be so pronounced that the individual has no recollection of the night before. This memory gap is also known as a "blackout". In addition, thinking and communication become so disorganized that the alcohol using individual may have difficulty being understood by others.[153]

Long-term use effects are those that appear following repeated use of alcohol over a long period of time. With prolonged use of alcohol, the brains of alcoholics may develop lesions due to the toxic effects of alcohol and its breakdown products.[154] The organic brain disorders that are a consequence of the prolonged and heavy use of alcohol are at times irreversible.

Pertaining to learning and memory capabilities, research conducted at Middlesex Hospital in London with identical twins where one sibling was a drinker and the other not, revealed that drinking siblings scored much lower on every mental test administered than their sober counterparts. In addition, the longer the duration of alcohol consumption by one twin, the lower the test score reported.[155] Portnoff found that individuals who began drinking in their teens appeared to have more cognitive impairment than those who began drinking later in adult years.[156] Researchers have also revealed that cognitive skills remained weak even after abstinence, suggesting permanent impairment due to chronic alcohol abuse.[157] In regard to alcohol use and educational deficiency, studies have shown that moderate levels of alcohol consumption can result in impaired learning and memory deficits.[158] Heavy drinking can seriously and, at times irreversibly, alter the intellectual functioning of the individual.[159] Alcohol use and abuse has also been found to diminish academic competitiveness, impair academic performance, devalue role and importance of education, lead to increased absenteeism, and impede social skills and emotional skills.[160]

The Diagnostic and Statistical Manual of Mental Disorders-III-R (DSM-III-R) describes several alcohol-induced organic mental disorders.[161]

Alcohol Intoxication is defined as a recent ingestion of alcohol with maladaptive behavioral changes, "e.g., disinhibition of sexual or aggressive impulses, mood lability, impaired judgment, impaired social or occupational functioning." Complications that ensue with alcohol intoxication are accidents, homicides, and suicides (these are discussed in greater detail in Chapter 3 "Alcohol and Adverse Social Consequences").

Alcohol Hallucinosis is a disorder in which the individual experiences vivid and persistent visual or auditory hallucinations shortly after stopping alcohol ingestion, usually within 48 hours. This disorder may be experienced by an individual who is considered Alcohol Dependent. This disorder also may be confused with Schizophrenia if an inadequate evaluation or history is taken of the individual.

Alcohol Amnestic Disorder is a vitamin deficiency associated with prolonged and heavy ingestion of alcohol. This disorder is also known as Korsakoff's Syndrome or Korsakoff's Psychosis. Korsakoff's Psychosis is characterized by profound confusion, disorientation, general fatigue, apathy, amnesiac confabulation, hallucinations, depression, and anxiety.[162,163] Confabulation is the attempt to fill in memory gaps by creating stories that may change from minute to minute without the individual realizing it.[164]

Korsakoff's Psychosis is part of a continuum of pathological changes known as Wernicke-Korsakoff Syndrome that take place in the brain after prolonged ingestion of alcohol. Wernicke Syndrome or Wernicke's encephalopathy refers to alcohol-related brain degeneration and is characterized by confusion, nystagmus (involuntary rapid horizontal eye movements) which can lead to eye paralysis, and loss of muscle coordination.[165] Wernicke's Syndrome can be treated with Vitamin B1 (thiamine) therapy. However, Wernicke-Korsakoff's syndrome has been reported to be irreversible in approximately 25 percent of individuals.[166] McEvoy reports that in patients diagnosed with Wernicke-Korsakoff syndrome, 20 percent recover completely, 60 percent show improvement, 20 percent require permanent institutionalization.[167] If Wernicke's Syndrome is not attended to, Korsakoff's psychosis will appear and Korsakoff's psychosis is not reversible.

In those individuals that do not develop Korsakoff's psychosis, cortical atrophy is prevalent and may be responsible for cognitive changes including deficits in visuospatial functions or the inability to deal with objects on a two-dimensional or three-dimensional level.[168-170]

The **DSM-III-R** describes Dementia associated with alcoholism as a disorder following prolonged and heavy ingestion of alcohol.[171] Whereas patients diagnosed with Korsakoff's psychosis retain normal intelligence but exhibit disabling behavioral problems and memory deficits, patients with Alcoholic Dementia have an overall decline in intellectual functioning in addition to memory loss.[172]

The individual diagnosed with alcohol related dementia experiences an impairment in abstract thinking, difficulty in defining words and concepts, impaired judgment, aphasia (disorder of language), apraxia (inability to carry out motor activities despite intact comprehension and motor function), agnosia (inability to recognize or identify objects), and inability to visualize on a three-dimensional level.[173] Only 10 percent of these patients are reported to show improvement of symptoms after prolonged abstinence. Dementia associated with alcoholism is the second most common adult dementia after Alzheimer's.[174,175]

In regard to Alzheimer's Disease, Liss reported that ingestion of alcohol plays a role in the acceleration of the Alzheimer disease process. Based on autopsy findings, the incidence of Alzheimer's disease was found in over 80 percent of those individuals with a history of serious alcohol abuse. In many of those cases a coexisting alcoholic encephalopathy was also present.[176]

16. Alcohol and Seizures

Hauser and colleagues reported that newly diagnosed cases of epilepsy have no risk factors other than a history of alcohol abuse.[177] In studies of diagnosed epileptics who on occasion ingest alcohol, seizure occurrence was associated with their drinking.[178] In addition, epileptics who drink to intoxication increase their risk factors due to the interaction of alcohol and anti-convulsant medication by either reducing the effectiveness of their medication or the medication producing potentially dangerous side effects. In general, physicians should be aware of their patients diagnosed with epilepsy who drink alcohol.

17. Alcohol and AIDS

AIDS or Acquired Immune Deficiency Syndrome is a disease that damages the body's immune system or the body's ability to fight off serious infections and illnesses.[179] AIDS is the end stage of a viral infection caused by the human immunodeficiency virus (HIV) and is characterized by a defect in natural immunity against disease. Individuals who have AIDS are susceptible to illnesses which would not be a threat to anyone with a normally functioning immune system. It is believed that alcohol abuse in HIV infected individuals may accelerate the progression of AIDS. Although at this time there is no substantial data verifying that theory, the New York State Division of Alcohol and Alcohol Abuse lists five reasons why alcohol abuse may indeed play a role in HIV infection and progression into AIDS. The reasons outlined are as follows:

"- It (alcohol abuse) decreases the number of white blood cells, which make up a significant portion of the immune system.
- It causes liver disease, which inhibits the body's ability to form T-cells, the white blood cells targeted by HIV.
- It often leads to a decrease in the number of T-cells and to poor health.
- It results in stress, which harms immune functioning.
- It can be toxic to bone marrow and the spleen"[180]

The AIDS Institute in New York has identified that both alcohol and cocaine suppress the immune system and speed up the process of the HIV virus.[181] Furthermore, MacGregor outlined four major immune defense systems which are adversely affected by chronic alcohol abuse.[182]

1. Antibody production is affected in the presence of alcohol.
2. The production of polymorphonuclear leukocytes (bacteria devouring cells) is

decreased in the bone marrow by chronic alcohol consumption. This effect is reversed once the person abstains from alcohol.

3. The reticuloendothelial system is impaired. This system produces macrophages (cells found in loose connective tissues and various organs of the body) necessary for the removal of bacteria. The reticuloendothelial cells eliminate worn out cells, especially red blood cells, and function in the repair of injured tissue.

4. T-cells, specialized white cells which destroy viruses or tumor cells, are reduced in the circulation. The reduction of T-cells permits the development of diseases to which the individual has no immunity to.

Once the person has an impaired immune system, he/she is exposed to life-threatening illnesses and diseases. One of the most common opportunistic infections diagnosed in AIDS patients is a form of pneumonia called pneumocystis carinii pneumonia. MacGregor reported that pneumonia is more likely to occur in alcoholics than in nondrinkers; and death from pneumonia is three times greater in chronic alcohol abusers than in the non-drinking population.[183] Therefore, the chronic alcoholic, with a suppressed immune system, may be more vulnerable to HIV infections and AIDS, including forms of pneumonia, toxoplasmosis of the brain, or Kaposi's Sarcoma (a form of cancer that arises in the skin).

In regard to youth, sexually transmitted diseases, and AIDS, Goldsmith identified that heterosexual transmission of AIDS is two to three times greater among adolescents than among adults.[184] In a review of research pertaining to adolescents, Leigh and Morrison revealed that although it is difficult to discern a causal relationship, youth who are sexually active are more likely to use alcohol and a positive correlation exists between alcohol use and adolescent sexual activity.[185] In addition, researchers have pointed out that adolescents who drink and engage in sexual activity are less likely to use condoms or contraceptives as compared with nondrinking sexually active teens.[186-188] Leigh and Morrison have concluded that the use of alcohol is associated with early sexual activity and may be due to societal acceptance of alcohol as a sexual disinhibitor.[189] Therefore, as long as sexual activity and the use of alcohol is an accepted "rite of passage" among adolescents, risk-taking behaviors in the form of unprotected sex will leave youth vulnerable to STD's and AIDS.

SUMMARY

Alcohol abuse is directly related to one-third of all deaths in the United States and either contributes to or causes many diseases or illnesses. The following is a summary of the adverse physical complications caused by alcohol abuse:
- Cancer of the mouth, tongue, pharynx, larynx, esophagus, colon, rectum, pancreas, breast.
- Esophagitis
- Gastritis
- Mallory-Weiss Syndrome
- Ulcers
- Pancreatitis
- Alcoholic Fatty Liver
- Alcoholic Hepatitis
- Cirrhosis
- Heart Disease
- Arrhythmias
- Endocarditis
- Cardiac Fibrillation
- Cardiomyopathy
- Alcoholic Myopathy
- Osteoporosis
- Osteopemia
- Idiopathic Osteonecrosis
- Increase in average blood cell size
- Anemia

- Decreased white blood cells
- Hypoglycemia
- Hyperlipidemia
- Hypertension
- Stroke
- Pneumococcal pneumonia
- Aspirative pneumonia
- Gonadal and adrenal effects
- Korsakoff's Syndrome
- Wernicke-Korsakoff Syndrome
- Cortical Atrophy
- Acceleration of Alzheimer's Disease
- Acceleration of AIDS

The tragic reality of the consequences of alcohol abuse is that many of the preceding physical complications are completely preventable. No, abstention from alcohol will not prevent illnesses from other causes; e.g. hypertension due to smoking or poor dietary habits. However, abstention from alcohol may prevent these illnesses when no other predisposing factors exist. Furthermore, alcohol abuse often is the sole contributing factor to such illnesses as Alcoholic Hepatitis, Alcoholic Cirrhosis, Alcoholic Myopathy or Korsakoff's Syndrome. It is clear that many of the life threatening consequences of alcohol abuse are directly linked to the toxic effects of alcohol ingestion. Abstention from alcohol often means prevention of disabling conditions.

REFERENCES

1. Fox, V., Conway, J. P., and Schweigler, J., Alcoholism, in **Handbook of Severe Disabilities**, Clowers, S., Ed., U.S. Government Printing Office, Washington, D.C., 1982, chap. 17.

2. Spence, W. R., **The Medical Consequences of Alcoholism**, Health Edco, Waco, Texas, 1987.

3. Gloeckner, C., From drinking to disease, **Current Health, 17**, 23, 1990.

4. Jacobs, M. R. and Fehr, K. O., Rev. Eds., **Drugs and Drug Abuse: A Reference Text**, 2nd Ed., Addiction Research Foundation, Toronto, Canada, 1987.

5. Gloeckner, **From drinking**, 1990.

6. Spence, **The Medical**, 1987.

7. Wynder, E. L., Toward the prevention of laryngeal cancer, **Laryngoscope, 85**, 1190, 1975.

8. Sporn, M. B., Dunlop, N. M., Newton, D. L., and Smith, J. M., Prevention of chemical carcinogenesis by vitamin A and its synthetic analogs (retinoids), **Federation Proceedings, 35**(6), 1332, 1976.

9. Wynder, E. L. and Chan, P. C., The possible role of riboflavin deficiency in epithelial neoplasia. II. Effect on skin tumor development, **Cancer, 26**, 1221, 1970.

10. Boyles, S., Alcohol risk in oral cancers may be topical, **Cancer Weekly, 4**, April 29, 1991.

11. Moore, M. H. and Gerstein, D. R., Eds., **Alcohol and Public Policy: Beyond the Shadow of Prohibition**, National Academy Press, Washington, D. C., 1981.

12. Rothman, K. H., Cann, C. I., and Fried, M. P., Carcinogenicity of dark liquor, **The American Journal of Public Health, 79**, 1516, 1989.

13. Edell, D., Smoking, drinking and nose sprays, **Edell Health Letter, 8**, 5, August 1989.

14. Wynder, **Possible**, 1970.

15. Beer consumption increases oral cancer risk, **NCI Cancer Weekly, 16**, August 20, 1990.

16. Moore, **Alcohol**, 1981.

17. Nelson, D. J., Group helps smokers break addictive cycle, **Minneapolis Star Tribune, VIII**(53), 8, 1989.

18. Boyles, **Cancer**, 1991.

19. Boyles, **Cancer**, 1991.
20. Gloeckner, **From drinking**, 1990.
21. Larkin, M., Nutrient snatchers: It isn't only our vices that can rob our bodies of vitamins and minerals, **Mature Health**, 24, November 1989.
22. Spence, **The Medical**, 1987.
23. Diet and esophageal cancer, **Nutrition Research, 43**, April 1990.
24. La Veccia, C. and Negri, E., The role of alcohol in esophageal cancer in non-smokers, and of tobacco in non-drinkers, **NCI Cancer Weekly, 23**, July 10, 1989.
25. Mezey, E., Alcohol abuse and digestive diseases, **Alcohol Health and Research World, 10**(2), 6, 1985/86.
26. Shirazi, S. S. and Platz, C. E., Effect of alcohol on canine esophageal mucosa, **Journal of Surgical Research, 25**, 373, 1978.
27. Spence, **The Medical**, 1987.
28. Mezey, **Alcohol**, 1985/86.
29. Gottfried, E. B., Korsten, M. A., and Lieber, C. S., Gastritis and duodenitis induced by alcohol: An endoscopic and histologic assessment (abstract). **Gastroenterology, 70**, A-32, 1976.
30. Mendoza, T., Very distant relatives: Alcohol and nutrition, **Current Health, 20**, October 2, 1990.
31. Radcliffe, A., Rush, P., Sites, C. F., and Cruse, J. **Pharmer's Almanac: Pharmacology of Drugs**, MAC Publishing, Denver, Colorado, 1989.
32. Mezey, **Alcohol**, 1985/86.
33. Mendoza, **Very distant**, 1990.
34. Willoughby, A., **The Alcohol Troubled Person: Known and Unknown**, Nelson-Hall, Chicago, Illinois, 1984.
35. Doweiko, H. E., **Concepts of Chemical Dependency, Brooks**, Cole, Pacific Grove, California, 1990.
36. Gottfried, **Gastritis**, 1976.
37. Spence, **The Medical**, 1987.
38. Doweiko, **Concepts**, 1990.

39. Mendoza, **Very distant**, 1990.
40. Radcliffe, **Pharmer's**, 1989.
41. National Institute on Alcohol Abuse and Alcoholism (NIAAA), Medical consequences of alcohol. Special Focus: The fifth special report to the U. S. Congress on alcohol and health, **Alcohol Health and Research World, 9**(1), 19, 1984.
42. Schuckit, M. A., **Drug and Alcohol Abuse: A Clinical Guide to Diagnosis and Treatment**, 2nd Ed., Plenum Press, New York, 1984.
43. Is alcohol a risk? **Executive Health Report, 6**, April 1989.
44. Hirayama, T., Association between alcohol consumption and cancer of the sigmoid colon: Observations from a Japanese cohort study, **The Lancet,** II(8665), 725, September 23, 1989.
45. Korsten, **Role**, 1990.
46. Radcliffe, **Pharmer's**, 1989.
47. Nace, E. P., **The Treatment of Alcoholism**, Brunner/Mazel, New York, 1987.
48. Korsten, **Role**, 1990.
49. NIAAA, **Medical**, 1984.
50. Olsen, G. W., Mandel, J. S., Gibson, R. W., Wattenberg, L. W., and Schuman, L. M., A case-control study of pancreatic cancer and cigarettes, alcohol, coffee and diet, **The American Journal of Public Health, 79**, 1061, August 1989.
51. Farrow, D. C. and Davis, S., Risk of pancreatic cancer in relation to medical history and the use of tobacco, alcohol and coffee, **International Journal on Cancer, 45**(5), 816, May 15, 1990.
52. Rubin, E., How alcohol damages the body, **Alcohol Health and Research World, 13**(4), 322, 1989.
53. Arria, A. M., Tarter, R. E., and Van Thiel, D. H., Liver-brain relations in alcoholics. Special focus: Alcohol and the brain. **Alcohol Health and Research World, 14**, 112, 1990.
54. Nace, **The Treatment**, 1987.

55. Arria, **Liver**, 1990.
56. Spence, **The Medical**, 1987.
57. Ray, O. and Ksir, C., **Drugs, Society and Human Behavior**, Times Mirror/Mosby, St. Louis, Missouri, 1987.
58. Arria, **Liver**, 1990.
59. Nace, **The Treatment**, 1987.
60. Arria, **Liver**, 1990.
61. Nace, **The Treatment**, 1987.
62. Ray, **Drugs**, 1987.
63. Nace, **The Treatment**, 1987.
64. Ray, **Drugs**, 1987.
65. Jacobs, **Drugs**, 1987.
66. National Institute of Diabetes and Digestive and Kidney Diseases (NIDDKD), **Cirrhosis of the Liver, NIH # 92-1134**, National Digestive Diseases Information Clearinghouse, Bethesda, Maryland, November, 1991.
67. Ray, **Drugs**, 1987.
68. Spence, **The Medical**, 1987.
69. Rubin, **How**, 1989.
70. Podolsky, D. M., NIAAA minority research activities, **Alcohol Health and Research World, 11**(2), 4, 1986/87.
71. Radcliffe, **Pharmer's**, 1989.
72. Ray, **Drugs**, 1987.
73. Radcliffe, **Pharmer's**, 1989.
74. NIDDKD, **Cirrhosis**, 1991.
75. Nace, **The Treatment**, 1987.
76. Rothschild, M. A., Oratz, M. and Schreiber, S. S., Alcohol-induced liver disease; does nutrition play a role? **Alcohol Health and Research World, 13,** 228, 1989.
77. NIAAA, **Medical**, 1984.
78. Doweiko, **Concepts**, 1990.
79. Davidson, D. M., Cardiovascular effects of Alcohol, **The Western Journal of Medicine, 151**, 430, October 1989.
80. Napier, K., Alcohol ad the heart - a loaded question, **Solutions for Better Health, 20**, 1990.
81. Radcliffe, **Pharmer's**, 1989.
82. Regan, T. J., Alcohol and the cardio-

vascular system, **The Journal of the American Medical Association, 264**, 377, July 18, 1990.
83. Davidson, **Cardiovascular**, 1989.
84. Koskinen, P., Kupari, M., and Leinonen, H., Role of alcohol in recurrences of atrial fibrillation in persons less than 65 years of age, **American Journal of Cardiology, 66**, 954, October 15, 1990.
85. Regan, **Alcohol**, 1990.
86. NIAAA, **Medical**, 1984.
87. Regan, **Alcohol**, 1990.
88. Rubin, **How**, 1989.
89. Rubin, **How**, 1989.
90. NIAAA, **Medical**, 1984.
91. Nace, **The Treatment**, 1987.
92. Rubin, **How**, 1989.
93. Urbano-Marquez, A., Estruch, R., Navarro-Lopez, F., Grau, J. M., Mont, L., and Rubin, E., The effects of alcoholism on skeletal and cardiac muscle, **New England Journal of Medicine, 320**(7), 409, 1989.
94. Rubin, **How**, 1989.
95. Mendoza, **Very distant**, 1990.
96. Rubin, **How**, 1989.
97. Nace, **The Treatment**, 1987.
98. NIAAA, **Medical**, 1984.
99. Radcliffe, **Pharmer's**, 1989.
100. Edell, D., Heavy drinking weakens muscles, **Edell Health Letter, 8**, 1, June 1989.
101. NIAAA, **Medical**, 1984.
102. Bliven, F. E., The skeletal system: Alcohol as a factor, in **Encyclopedia Handbook of Alcoholism**, E. M. Pattison and E. Kaufman, Eds., pp. 215, Gardner Press, New York, 1982.
103. Nace, **The Treatment**, 1987.
104. Radcliffe, **Pharmer's**, 1989.
105. NIAAA, **Medical**, 1984.
106. Unger, K. W. and Johnson, D., Red blood cell mean corpuscular volume: A potential indicator of alcohol usage in a working population, **American Journal of the Medical Sciences, 267**, 281, 1974.
107. Nace, **The Treatment**, 1987.
108. Radcliffe, **Pharmer's**, 1989.

109. Nace, **The Treatment**, 1987.
110. NIAAA, **Medical**, 1984.
111. Gloeckner, **From..**, 1990.
112. Radcliffe, **Pharmer's**, 1989.
113. Gloeckner, **From..**, 1990.
114. Gloeckner, **From..**, 1990.
115. Radcliffe, **Pharmer's**, 1989.
116. Alcohol and blood pressure: United States and Japan, **Nutrition Research Newsletter, 29**, March 1991.
117. Gloeckner, **From..**, 1990.
118. Witteman, J. C. M., Willett, W. C., Stampfer, M. J., Colditz, G. A., Kok, F. J., Sacks, F. M., Speizer, F. E., Rosner, B., and Hennekens, C. H., Relation of moderate alcohol consumption and risk of systemic hypertension in women, **American Journal of Cardiology, 65**(9), 633, March 1, 1990.
119. Hudnall, M., Alcohol poses many health risks, few benefits, **Environmental nutrition, 12**(2), 1, July 1989.
120. Davidson, **Cardiovascular**, 1989.
121. Hudnall, **Alcohol**, 1989.
122. Napier, **Alcohol**, 1990.
123. Ray, **Drugs**, 1987.
124. Regan, **Alcohol**, 1990.
125. Spence, **The Treatment**, 1987.
126. Doweiko, **Concepts**, 1990.
127. Spence, **The Treatment**, 1987.
128. Cramer, S. L., Alcoholism and bullous changes of the lungs, **Alcohol Health and Research World**, 13, 166, 1989.
129. Cramer, **Alcoholism**, 1989.
130. Peterson, C. M., Mix alcohol, high blood glucose and you can create havoc, **Diabetes in the News, 9**, 33, 1990.
131. Peterson, **Mix**, 1990.
132. NIAAA, **Medical**, 1984.
133. Ben, G., Gnudi, L., Maran, A., Gigante, A., Duner, E., Iori, E., Tiengo, A., and Avogaro, A., Effects of chronic alcohol intake on carbohydrate and lipid metabolism in subjects with type II (non-insulin dependent) diabetes. **American Journal of Medicine, 90**,

70, 1991.

134. Van Thiel, D. H. and Lester, R., The effect of chronic alcohol abuse on sexual function, **Clinics in Endocrinology and Metabolism, 8,** 499, 1979.

135. Van Thiel, D. H., Gonadal effects, **Gastroenterology, 81,** 608, 1981.

136. Rubin, **How,** 1989.

137. Van Thiel, D. H. and Chiao, Y. B., Biochemical mechanisms that contribute to alcohol-induced hypogonadism in the male, **Alcoholism: Clinical and Experimental Research, 7,** 131, 1983.

138. Gavaler, J. S., Effects of alcohol on endocrine function in post-menopausal women; a review, **Journal of Studies on Alcohol, 46**(6), 495, 1985.

139. Mendelson, J. H., Mello, N. K., Teoh, S. K., and Ellingboe, J., Alcohol effects on plasma estradiol levels following LHRH administration to women, in **Problems of Drug Dependence 1989: Proceedings of the 51st Annual Scientific Meeting,** Harris, L. S., Ed., NIDA Research Monograph 95, 425, National Institute on Drug Abuse, Rockville, Maryland, 1989.

140. Teoh, S. K., Lex, B. W., Cochin, J., Mendelson, J. H., and Mello, N. K., Anterior pituitary, gonadal and adrenal hormones in women with alcohol and poly-drug abuse, in **Problems of Drug Dependence 1989: Proceedings of the 51st Annual Scientific Meeting,** Harris, L. S., Ed., NIDA Research Monograph 95, 425, National Institute on Drug Abuse, Rockville, Maryland, 1989.

141. Van Thiel, D. H. and Lester, R., The effect of chronic alcohol abuse on sexual function. **Clinics in Endocrinology and Metabolism, 8,** 499, 1979.

142. NIAAA, **Medical,** 1984.

143. Podolsky, D. M., Alcohol consumption and the risk of breast cancer, **Alcohol Health and Research World, 10**(3), 40, 1986.

144. Alcohol link to breast cancer

confirmed, **Nutrition Health Review, 4,** Spring 1989.
145. Boyles, **Alcohol,** 1991.
146. Young, T. B., Alcohol and breast cancer, **Nutrition Research Newsletter, 8,** September, 1989.
147. Hudnall, **Alcohol,** 1989.
148. Rosenberg, L., Slone, D., Shapiro, S., Kaufman, D. W., Helmrich, S., Miettinen, O. S., Stolley, P.D., Levy, M., Rosenshein, N. B., Schottenfeld, D., and Engle, R. L., Breast cancer and alcohol beverage consumption, **Lancet, 2,** 626, 1982.
149. Allen, R. P., Faillace, L. A., and Reynolds, D. M., Recovery of mental functioning in alcoholics following prolonged alcohol intoxication, **Journal of Nervous Mental Disorders, 153,** 417, 1971.
150. Jacobs, **Drugs,** 1987.
151. Long, J. A. and McLachlin, J. F. C., Abstract reasoning and perceptual-motor efficiency in alcoholics - impairment and reversibility, **Quarterly Journal of Studies in Alcoholism, 35,** 1220, 1974.
152. Rubin, **How,** 1989.
153. Jacobs, **Drugs,** 1987.
154. Charness, M. E., Alcohol and the brain, **Alcohol Health and Research World, 14,** 85, 1990.
155. Edell, D., This is your brain on booze. Research at Middlesex Hospital, London on alcohol's effect on the brain, **The Edell Health Letter,** 1, June 1991.
156. Portnoff, L., Halstead-Reitan impairment in chronic alcoholics as a function of age of drinking onset, **Clinical Neuropsychology, 4,** 115, 1982.
157. Fein, G., Bachman, L., Fisher, S., and Davenport, L., Cognitive impairments in abstinent alcoholics, **The Western Journal of Medicine, 152,** 531, 1990.
158. Lister, R. G., Eckardt, M., and Weingartner, H., Ethanol intoxication and memory: Recent developments and new directions, in

Recent Developments in Alcoholism, Vol. V, Galanter, M., Ed., Plenum Press, New York, 1987.
159. Rubin, **How**, 1989.
160. Grant, D. and Moore, B., MIBCA (Minnesota Institute on Black Chemical Abuse) sponsored conference: Groundwork for future action, **Alcohol Health and Research World, 11**(2), 18, 1986/87.
161. American Psychiatric Association, **Diagnostic and Statistical Manual**, 3rd Ed. revised, (DSM-III-R), American Psychiatric Press, Washington, D. C. 1987.
162. Grant, M. and Ritson, B., **Alcohol - The Prevention Debate**, St. Martin's Press, New York, 1983.
163. Jacobs, **Drugs**, 1987.
164. Radcliffe, **Pharmer's**, 1989.
165. Berman, M. O., Severe brain dysfunction: Alcoholic Korsakoff's syndrome, **Alcohol Health and Research World, 14**, 120, 1990.
166. Dreyfus, P. M., Effects of alcohol on the nervous system, in **Fermented Food Beverages in Nutrition**, Vol. XXI, Gastieneau, C. F., Darby, W. J., and Turner, T. B., Eds., Academic Press, New York, 1979.
167. McEvoy, J. P., The chronic neuropsychiatric disorders associated with alcoholism, in **Encyclopedic Handbook of Alcoholism**, Pattison, E. M. and Kaufman, E., Eds., Gardner Press, New York, 1982.
168. Berman, **Severe**, 1990.
169. Lishman, W. A., Cerebral disorder in alcoholism: Syndromes of impairment, **Brain, 104**(1), 1, 1981.
170. Wilkinson, D. A. and Carlen, P. L., Morphological abnormalities in the brains of alcoholics: Relationship to age, psychological test scores and patient type, in **Alcoholism and Aging: Advances in Research**, Wood, W. G. and Elias, M. F., Eds., CRC Press, Boca Raton, Florida.

171. American Psychiatric Association, **DSM-III-R**, 1987.
172. Doria, J., Interview with Dr. Michael J. Eckardt, **Alcohol Health and Research World**, 349, 1989.
173. American Psychiatric Association, **DSM-III-R**, 1987.
174. Doria, **Interview**, 1989.
175. Nace, **The Treatment**, 1987.
176. Liss, L., Alcohol damage and Alzheimer's disease, **Alcoholism and Addiction Magazine, 8**, 53, April 1988.
177. Hauser, W. A., Ng, S. K. C., and Brust, J. C. M., Alcohol, seizures, and epilepsy, **Epilepsia, 29**(Suppl. 2), S66, 1988.
178. Stoil, M. J., Epilepsy, seizures and alcohol, **Alcohol Health and Research World, 13**, 138, 1989.
179. **AIDS and Drug Abuse**, Montefiore Medical Center, Bronx, New York, 1988.
180. Does alcohol accelerate AIDS progression? **AIDS Alert, 97**, June 1989.
181. AIDS Institute, New York State Department of Health (NYSDH), **HIV Counselor Training Manual**, NYSDH, New York, 1989.
182. Nace, **The Treatment**, 1987.
183. Nace, **The Treatment**, 1987.
184. Goldsmith, M. F., Stockholm speakers on adolescents and AIDS: "Catch them before they catch it", **Journal of the American Medical Association, 260**(6), 757, 1988.
185. Leigh, B. C. and Morrison, D. M., Alcohol consumption and sexual risk-taking in adolescents, **Alcohol Health and Research World, 15**(1), 58, 1991.
186. Flanagan, B. J. and Hitch, M. A., Alcohol use, sexual intercourse, and contraception: An exploratory study, **Journal of Alcohol and Drug Education, 31**(3), 6, 1986.
187. Hingson, R. W., Strunin, L., Berlin, B. M., and Heeren, T., Beliefs about AIDS, use of alcohol, drugs, and unprotected sex among Massachusetts adolescents, **American Journal of**

Public Health, **80**(3), 295, 1990.
   188. Robertson, J. A. and Plant, M. A., Alcohol, sex and risks of HIV infection, **Drug and Alcohol Dependence, 22**(1), 75, 1988.
   189. Leigh, **Alcohol**, 1991.

Chapter 3

ALCOHOL AND ADVERSE SOCIAL CONSEQUENCES

I. ACCIDENTS

According to the U.S. Department of Health and Human Services, alcohol has been implicated in four leading causes of accidents in the United States - motor vehicle crashes, falls, drownings, and fires.[1]

A. Traffic Accidents

In 1988 the Surgeon General's Workshop on Drunk Driving revealed that an estimated 2,000,000 drivers are arrested each year for driving under the influence of alcohol. With statistics this high, drunk driving continues to be one of the Nation's most serious public health problems. It is estimated that a traffic fatality occurs every 22 minutes. In addition to the fatalities, each year approximately 534,000 people incur injuries due to alcohol-related collisions, with an estimated 40,000 of these injuries being serious.[2] Alcohol related fatalities are three times more likely to occur at night than during the day. Seventy-seven percent of fatally injured drivers 25 years of age or older and who were intoxicated occurred on weekend nights in 1988.[3]

The National Highway Traffic Safety Administration defines an alcohol related fatality or car crash when the driver, pedestrian or bicyclist has an estimated blood alcohol concentration (BAC) of 0.01 percent or above. A BAC of 0.10 or greater is considered the legal limit in most states for intoxication.[4,5]

The National Accident Sampling System (NASS) of NHTSA collects data on alcohol-related injuries from motor vehicle accidents. Of the alcohol-involved traffic accidents in 1986, NASS reported that approxmately 50 percent resulted in minor to moderate injuries; whereas, 8 percent of alcohol-related crashes resulted in serious to severe injuries.[6] In a study conducted in a trauma center over a 28-month period, researchers found that out of 2,262 trauma patients, 93 percent had a blood alcohol level determination. Most of the trauma patients were male (75 percent) and most were injured in a motor vehicle accident (72 percent).[7]

Although the number of people killed in an alcohol-related crash where at least one participant had a BAC of 0.10 percent or greater decreased from 46 percent in 1982 to 39 percent in 1988, traffic crashes remain the greatest single cause of death for every age between five and 32 years.[8] Alcohol-related fatalities still remained high in this time frame among 25 to 34 year old drivers or among 20 to 60 year old pedestrians. In addition, alcohol use remained high among motorcycle drivers.[9]

Although statistics show that there is an apparent decline in alcohol-related car crashes, attention must be given to select populations where there is little reduction in alcohol use and traffic-related fatalities or injuries. The measure of alcohol still remains high in car accidents involving 18 to 24 year old drivers. Fifty-one percent of fatal accidents in January, February and March of 1990 comprising of 21 to 24 year olds, involved a driver who was legally drunk.[10] In research conducted with 18 men and 18 women between the ages of 18 and 25 years, it was noted that male subjects took more risks, drove more dangerously and, that peer attitudes played a role in drinking and driving.[11] This last statement supports the findings stated earlier in this section that most trauma patients hospitalized after a motor-vehicle accident were male.

In 1989 the prevalence of intoxication in fatal car crashes in drivers between the ages of 15 and 25 years increased with age: 15-71 years, 54 percent were intoxicated; 18-20 years old, 68 percent were intoxicated; 21-24 years old, 77 percent were intoxicated; and 25 years old, 79 percent were intoxicated.[12] Surgeon General Antonia Novello reported in June 1991, that one/third of all teenagers who drink also ride with friends who have been drinking despite the fact that they are aware of the dangers of drinking and driving.[13] Once again, it is apparent that peer attitudes play a dramatic role in the drinking and driving behaviors of youth between the ages of 13 and 25 years.

B. Alcohol Use and Flying

The National Traffic Safety Board reported that between 1975 and 1981, out of 4,947 fatal aviation accidents, 414 involved alcohol. In fact, almost 800 individuals lost their lives in aviation accidents in which a pilot was impaired due to alcohol.[14,15]

In a study conducted by Billings, NASA-Ames Research Center with air carrier pilot volunteers during simulated flights between San Francisco and Los Angeles, it was determined that errors increased linearly and significantly with increasing blood alcohol levels. The errors that increased were related to planning and performance, procedures and failures of vigilance. In fact, serious errors occurred even at the lowest blood alcohol level studied - 0.025% as compared with control values.[16]

Alcohol use is known to cause decreased motor control, and reduce pilot ability to process and integrate information. Heavy alcohol use also creates a distortion of balance. Sixteen percent of 2200 private and commercial pilots studied engaged in heavy drinking which can distort equilibrium.[17] Evidence was also found that coordination and visual-motor skills were impaired up to 14 hours after the pilot had consumed three to four alcoholic beverages.[18] In general, pilots were found to overestimate the level of alcohol needed to impair their performance.

Another effect of alcohol consumption on flying ability is the added effect of reduced oxygen. Researchers have found that the intoxicating effect of alcohol is magnified in the upper atmosphere and in an unpressurized aircraft. Therefore, the effect of two drinks at high altitudes is increased to the intoxication level of four drinks at ground level.[19]

C. Boating Accidents and Drownings

Drowning is the third leading cause of accidental death in the United States, and alcohol is implicated in approximately one-half of all deaths from drowning.[20,21] Studies published by the National Institute on Alcohol Abuse and Alcoholism and the National Council on Alcoholism have revealed that alcohol is a significant factor in as many as 65 to 68 percent of all drownings. The United States Coast Guard reported in 1984 that nine out of ten individuals who die in a boating accident do so by drowning. In a survey of 10,000 boat owners, it was revealed that 93 percent felt that alcohol abuse on boats is a problem and 46 percent felt that alcohol abuse on boats was a significant problem.[22]

One reason why alcohol is such a significant problem is that the elements (sun, wind, motion of the water) that boaters are exposed to are exacerbated by alcohol. In other words, a type of fatigue sets in most individuals who have been on the water for several hours. The use of alcohol during this time on the water compounds the effects and presents a potential hazard.[23]

The use of alcohol may contribute to boating and drowning accidents in the following ways:

a.) Bravado or risk taking increases with

alcohol intake, thereby decreasing one's ability to react properly with the result being a fall from watercraft, pier, bank, or pool. The loss of balance caused by alcohol ingestion is the most important factor in drownings.

b.) In swimming, alcohol hastens loss of body heat, contributes to psychomotor impairment and disorientation. Even in the best swimmer, alcohol interferes with the diving reflex and one's ability to hold a breath of air in the water.[24-26]

As in alcohol-related traffic fatalities, males appear more likely to be involved in aquatic accidents. A study conducted by the Boston University School of Public Health revealed that men were 12 times more likely than women to be involved in a boating accident that resulted in drowning and five times more likely to be involved in other types of drowning. The findings were attributed to the fact that men had a greater tendency to drink alcohol when involved in aquatic activities.[27]

D. Fires and Burns

The fourth leading cause of accidental death in the United States is attributable to fires and burns. Although no causal relationship can be suggested between alcohol and fires and burns, a number of studies have proposed that alcohol consumption is associated with increased risk of fires and burns.[28,29]

In a study conducted in the mid-sixties, it was indicated that 64 percent of individuals who died as a result of a fire had BACs greater or equal to 0.10 percent at the time of death.[30] A number of studies also revealed that alcohol consumption was more frequent among victims of cigarette fires suggesting that smoking and drinking increase the risk for fire and burn fatalities or injuries.[31] Twenty percent of the fires that claimed more than one individual were allegedly caused by a fire started by a cigarette dropped by an intoxicated smoker.[32] Furthermore, alcohol abusing individuals were 10 times more likely to die because of a fire.[33]

E. Falls
Alcohol increases the risk of falls and is the most common cause of nonfatal injuries.[34] Alcohol is also the second leading cause of fatal accidents.[35] Researchers asserted that alcoholics were five to 13 times more likely to die from falls as compared with non-alcohol abusing individuals.[36,37]

In a Center for Environmental Health report, alcohol use was found in 10 percent of 1,740 persons admitted to a hospital emergency room due to fall injuries in 1975. In addition, 22 percent of 78 individuals who sought treatment for repeated fall injuries were due to alcohol use.[38] In 1983, Honkanen and colleagues reported that of 313 individuals seeking emergency room treatment due to fall injuries, 60 percent had measurable BACs and 53 percent had BACs greater than 0.20 percent. Honkanen and colleagues concluded that individuals with BACs of 0.05 to 0.10 percent were three times at greater risk for suffering a fall and the risk increased with the BAC level. Individuals with BACs of 0.10 to 0.15 were 10 times at greater risk, and individuals with BACs of 0.16 or higher were 60 times at greater risk for experiencing a fall injury.[39]

F. Alcohol Use and Head Injuries
One of the most serious injuries that occurs as a result of alcohol intoxication is traumatic brain injury. Researchers have identified that alcohol abuse is the strongest predisposing element in traumatic brain injury.[40-43] In the general population, it

is estimated that approximately 325,000 cases of head injury occur annually in the United States. Contributing causes of traumatic brain injury in the general population are motor vehicle accidents (42%), falls (23%), and assaults (14%).[44] Approximately 50 percent of all traumatic brain injury is alcohol-related.[45]

It appears that the incidence of traumatic head injury in alcoholics is two to four times higher than in the general population.[46] Predisposition to traumatic brain injury was also found in individuals with a history of familial alcoholism. In fact, this risk appeared to be twice as high as in individuals without familial alcoholism.[47] (The impact of the alcoholic family is discussed in Chapter 6).

A survey conducted by the National Head Injury Foundation disclosed that before the brain injury occurred, approximately 55 percent of patients had some alcohol abuse problems and 40 percent had moderate to severe alcohol problems. Individuals with traumatic brain injury experience cognitive, behavioral and functional deficits. The following is a list of the possible impairments an individual with a head injury may face:[48,49]

-Disruption of short-term memory
-Confabulation (the attempt to fill in memory gaps by creating stories)
-Decreased insight
-Impaired abstract reasoning or the inability to integrate information
-Attention and concentration deficits
-Distractibility
-Personality changes
-Inappropriate social behaviors; such as impulsiveness or rude and aggressive behaviors
-Low tolerance for stress
-Emotional lability and broad mood swings
-Language and communication deficits
-Oral-motor difficulties

-Dysarthria (difficulty forming words)
-Aphasia (language disorder)
-Sensory deficits
-Visual-perceptual problems
-Impaired writing and reading abilities
-Tinnitus (ringing in the ears)
-Problem-solving difficulties
-Undefined or unrealistic goal setting.

Not surprisingly, all these impairments caused by brain injury are the same as those caused by alcohol intoxication. In fact, very often the intoxicated individual acts very much like the person who has experienced a traumatic brain injury; behaviors, motor functions and mental processes are all affected in similar ways.

Alcohol in the body at time of injury impairs the brain more acutely, and therefore, impedes and complicates medical outcome. Head trauma survivors with a pre-existing alcohol abuse history and intoxication at time of head injury experience slower and more difficult recoveries. One reason for a more difficult recovery is that alcohol is a central nervous system depressant and affects the body's ability to produce an appropriate response to hemorrhage and shock. Evidence based on animal studies conducted by J. Barth revealed that alcohol use before a head injury resulted in a higher incidence of cerebral hemorrhage. Furthermore, elevated blood alcohol levels at time of head injury pose a higher anesthesia risk for emergency surgery due to the synergistic effect of alcohol mixing with an anesthetic. Both alcohol and anesthetics are central nervous system depressants. Combining alcohol and anesthesia compounds the risk for a successful medical outcome.[50]

Further research has revealed that individuals intoxicated at the time of head injury had longer periods of coma and agitation. Lower cognitive status upon discharge was also noted. There appears to be a clear relationship between intoxication at time of head injury and lower cognitive performance and longer post-traumatic amnesia.[51] In addition, since the alcohol abusing individual's nutrition is often inadequate, he/she is predisposed to post-injury infection and impaired healing.[52] Long-term effects of alcohol ingestion also handicap the immune system and slow down the recovery process.[53]

In the rehabilitation process of the head injured person, it is imperative to take into consideration the patient's alcohol history as well as his/her familial alcohol history. Successful rehabilitation without this important component is doomed to failure. Alcohol education and counseling must be an integral part of the traumatic head injury rehabilitation process because the person who has experienced a head injury is much more susceptible to the adverse effects of alcohol, particularly cognitive effects. As with a head injury, alcohol affects the midbrain and frontal lobe regions that govern judgement, concentration and control impulses.[54]

Since alcohol dulls the perception, impairs judgement and interferes with mental processes in general, the individual is less able to compensate for cognitive deficits and is more likely to injure him/herself again. Clinicians have found that a second head injury is much worse. "One head injury plus one head injury does not equal two head injuries; the cumulative factor is more like three or four head injuries."[55] In addition, alcohol ingestion intensifies any problems the head injured individual may be experiencing with balance, memory or organization skills.

Unfortunately, Sparadeo and Gill reported that 54 percent of head injured individuals returned to using alcohol after their rehabilitation.[56] Among the reasons indicated for this recidivism are: 1.) boredom, 2.) emotional lability or physical difficulties, and 3.) lack of attention paid to the individual's need or desire to return to work, or not effectively preparing the individual for career change. However, boredom is the number one reason why an individual returns to drinking.[57] Therefore, head trauma rehabilitation programs must provide programs that teach alternative behaviors to drinking alcohol or using drugs to cope with stress or boredom. Vocational and recreational therapists must also be cognizant of the fact that the individual may be more prone to substance abuse if he/she is not provided with the appropriate behavioral techniques to cope with an altered lifestyle due to a traumatic brain injury.[58]

Based on this information, effective and successful rehabilitation of head injured patients must include alcohol education and counseling services. It is evident that a history of alcohol and/or drug abuse can seriously undermine an individual's progress in acute and post-acute rehabilitation facilities. Long-term follow-up must be an inherent part of the overall treatment plan to determine the individual's recovery from both traumatic brain injury and alcohol abuse. Premature termination of follow-up services may result in relapse and possibly a second brain injury.

G. Alcohol Use and Spinal Cord Injuries

Approximately 7,800 individuals suffer spinal cord injury (SCI) each year in the United States alone. Of all reported SCIs 46 percent are complete or the total loss of sensation or function, and 54 percent are incomplete or resulting in partial loss. Quadriplegia and paraplegia occur in both categories.[59] But SCI involves more than the inability to move and experience loss of sensations, SCI patients also experience bowel and bladder impairment and loss of sexual functions.

Researchers have reported that 68 percent of all disabling SCIs were the result of alcohol and/or drug use at the time of injury.[60] Since drinking increases risk taking behaviors, impaired judgment due to alcohol use and abuse was a contributing factor to the accident that resulted in SCI.[61]

A disturbing factor regarding alcohol related SCI, is the fact that studies have revealed that alcohol abuse continues in a high percentage of clients with SCIs. The prevalence of alcohol use and abuse among SCI persons was reported between 49 percent and 62 percent after the onset of SCI.[62,63] Heinemann and colleagues have stressed that "persons with addiction problems who incur traumatic injury have special needs that require close collaboration of alcoholism treatment and rehabilitation medicine professionals."[64] As with traumatic brain injury, exclusion of alcoholism treatment plans or counseling with SCI clients will result in recidivism of alcohol problems and contribute to other physical and mental disorders.

All too often alcohol-related problems among the physically impaired have been ignored and a great deal of time, money and energy has been spent on the "symptoms" of alcohol problems that have resulted in physical impairment.[65,66] Greater attention needs to be focused on prevention of alcohol-related disabilities along with intervention and treatment of alcohol abuse and dependence issues with the person who incurred a disability as a result of alcohol use and abuse.

II. ALCOHOL, CRIME AND VIOLENCE

It has long been the contention of many researchers and practitioners that alcohol consumption may predispose an individual to violent behavior.[67,68] Researchers have noted that individuals who engage in criminal activity are more likely to have alcohol abuse problems. Despite the fact that no direct causal relationship between alcohol and crime has been established, studies have shown that 86 percent of those involved in assaults were intoxicated at the time of the injury.[69] In addition, studies of police reports and arrested populations identified that alcohol was present in 66 percent of all cases.[70] A literature review of 28 studies indicated that the majority of both victims of crime and offenders had been drinking alcohol prior to the crime committed.[71] In general, the higher the level of intoxication, the greater the severity and number of injuries sustained in either an assault or violent behavior.

In 1983, a national study was conducted by the Census Bureau for the U. S. Bureau of Justice Statistics, U. S. Department of Justice. The survey, conducted in local jails, pertained to the inmates' consumption of alcohol prior to the crime for which they were sentenced. The following are the findings of this survey.[72]

- Forty-eight percent of the inmates surveyed had been drinking prior to the crime.
- Fifty-four percent admitted to drinking for five or more hours before committing the crime.
- Fifty-four percent of the inmates sentenced for a violent crime consumed alcohol before the crime.
- Sixty-eight percent of those convicted of manslaughter reported drinking prior to the crime.
- Sixty-two percent of those convicted of assault admitted to consuming alcohol prior to the crime.
- Forty-nine percent of those convicted of murder or attempted murder reported consuming alcohol prior to the crime.
- Fifty-two percent of those convicted of

rape or sexual assault had been drinking alcohol prior to the crime. In regard to rape, several studies have suggested that individuals who commit rape are disproportionately apt to have been drinking before the rape or sexual assault took place.[73]

Furthermore, researchers have identified that paranoia and violence were connected with heavy alcohol use; as were increased aggressive and confrontive behaviors among young males who consumed alcohol on a regular basis.[74,75] In regard to adolescent males, there appeared to be a significant association between chronic alcohol consumption and violent crime.[76] Sixty-five percent of juveniles who committed serious crimes abused alcohol, whereas 85 percent who committed less severe offenses drank alcohol prior to the criminal act. Although alcohol was strongly linked with juvenile offenses, alcohol consumption was the strongest single predictor of criminal activity among black youth.[77]

A. Alcohol and Family Violence

The concept of abuse or family violence has defied easy definition. Lystad defined violence or abuse in the family as any "behavior that involves the direct use of physical aggression against household members which is against their will and detrimental to their growth potential. This includes behaviors of homicide, beatings and forced sex."[78] What causal factor alcohol plays in family violence has not been clearly established; however, excessive alcohol consumption in the family has been associated with various degrees of emotional and physical abuse. Researchers have reported that alcohol abuse and family violence frequently occur in the same families.[79,80] Estimated percentages of alcohol abuse occurring in families where domestic violence has been experienced have ranged from 25 to 30 percent, to as high as 80 percent.[81,82] Although alcohol abuse does not cause family violence, it has been postulated that it does exacerbate violence. Alcohol has been identified with disrupted family functioning as evidenced in the remarkably high rate of separation and divorce; seven times greater than that of the general population.[83]

Alcoholism has also been identified as a contributing factor in 40 percent of family court cases, and has been reported in 17 to 35 percent of divorces that involve violence.[84,85] In addition to high divorce rates among alcoholics, alcohol abuse also contributes to spouse abuse and child abuse.

1. **Spouse Abuse**

In a literature review, Hamilton and Collins cited excessive alcohol consumption in 45 to 60 percent of all cases of spouse abuse.[86] A telephone survey of more than 5,000 families in the United States revealed that drinking, social status and approval of violence were associated with high rates of wife abuse.[87] High rates of physical violence directed toward a spouse was also found among alcohol abusers in a study randomly conducted with 1200 individuals.[88] Another study revealed that physically violent men were reported to have higher levels of alcohol abuse than a comparison group who used alcohol but were nonviolent.[89] Although no causal relationship may exist between spouse abuse and alcohol abuse, based on these findings it is apparent that alcohol abuse plays an important factor in physical violence.

2. **Child Abuse**

The term child abuse takes into account sexual abuse, incest, emotional and physical abuse, neglect and abandonment. In 1983, the U. S. Department of Health and Human Services reported that one in three individuals who abused a child had been drinking prior to the act of abuse. Approximately 17 percent of all reported cases of child abuse have involved alcoholism.[90] A recent study reported that child abuse and alcohol problems are clearly associated. Randomly conducted interviews found that female alcoholics were more likely to abuse their children. The study also indicated that individuals who abuse their children were also more likely to abuse their spouses.[91]

In terms of long-term impact of abuse on the child, studies have revealed that children from alcoholic families exhibit emotional and behavioral problems.[92] Furthermore, children that either experience violence directly or are witnesses to family violence in an alcoholic home, are at greater risk for developing psychological problems.[93,94] After conducting laboratory studies and field investigations, researchers concluded that children exposed to anger reacted with various signs of distress which ranged from crying to acts of aggression.[95,96]

The most significant aspect of being a victim or witnessing an act of aggression toward a family member is the following: The threat of physical harm, whether personal or toward a family member, provokes the most intense of human reactions and leaves an emotional imprint, which often lasts a lifetime.[97,98] This emotional imprint may manifest itself as post-traumatic stress disorder and is more severe when the stressor is of human design.[99]

Often the difference between the child who was a direct victim of abuse as compared with the child who witnessed abusive behaviors is in the subsequent psychopathology manifested by the child. Whereas the "victim" may have dissociative symptoms which encompass psychogenic amnesia (a sudden failure to recall important personal events and is not due to an organic disturbance), the "witness" has full recall of the distressing event.[100] Despite this alleged difference between victims of abuse and witnesses to abuse, children who experience severe emotional, physical or sexual abuse (directly or indirectly) may manifest symptoms of post-traumatic stress disorder due to the intensity and duration of the abusive behaviors exhibited in the alcoholic family.

Post-traumatic stress disorder is defined by the **DSM-III-R** as follows:

"The essential feature of this disorder is the development of characteristic symptoms following a psychologically distressing event that is outside the range of usual human experience (i.e., outside the range of such common experiences as simple bereavement, chronic illness, business losses, and marital conflict). The stressor producing this syndrome would be markedly distressing to almost anyone, and is usually experienced with intense fear, terror, and helplessness. The characteristic symptoms involve reexperiencing the traumatic event, avoidance of stimulii associated with the event or numbing of general responsiveness and increased arousal."[101]

In life history interviews conducted with 18 women who were raised in alcoholic families, 15 women reported episodes of violence. These women, who were between the ages of 19 and 58 and of various educational and social backgrounds, were either the victims of beatings, sexual molestations, severe emotional abuse, or had witnessed acts of violence. All fifteen women related stories pertaining to the long-term impact of the alcoholic parent on their lives that bore a resemblance to characteristics of post-traumatic stress disorder as defined in the DSM-III-R.[102]

Although no causal relationship between

alcohol abuse and family violence has been established, it is clearly indicated by these studies that alcohol abuse does contribute to violence perpetrated on the spouse or child.

III. ALCOHOL ABUSE AND THE WORK ENVIRONMENT

Human disabilities may be caused by many factors. One of the primary factors or causes of debilitating illnesses or injuries which has received attention in recent years is in the area of environmental quality concerns. Environmental quality problems encompass a broad spectrum of recognized issues; e.g., water pollution, air pollution, toxic contamination, health and safety issues in the workplace, etc.[103] Health and safety issues in the workplace is in and of itself a broad category and many factors within the work environment may contribute to various causes of human disabilities; e.g. unsafe work areas leading to accidents.

How does alcohol abuse enter into this category of environmental concerns and, more specifically, the work environment? Since the 1970s considerable attention has been devoted to studying the impact of alcohol or drug abuse in the workplace. The impact of alcohol abuse on the part of a worker has far reaching consequences. For example, the continuum of the deleterious consequences of alcohol abuse in the workplace may run the gamut from excessive tardiness and absenteeism to conflicts with supervisors and co-workers to accidents on the job. Two factors, both cost related, are important to look at when dealing with alcohol abuse in the workplace. The first cost factor is the monetary or economic cost of dealing with an alcohol-abusing individual in the workplace. The second cost factor is the cost of a human life suffering the consequences of short-term or long-term alcohol abuse or dependence with the result being a physical or mental disability.

Unfortunately, the economic cost factor has taken precedence in assessing the impact of alcohol abuse on the workplace. However, despite the fact that monetary loss is the forerunner in analyzing alcohol abuse in the workplace, voluminous information does exist that points to the fact that the cost of human life as a result of alcohol abuse far outweighs the economic disadvantages to business and industry.

How extensive is the impact of alcohol abuse in the workplace? The Employee Assistance Professionals Association (EAPA) (formerly the Association of Labor-Management Administrators and Consultants on Alcoholism (ALMACA) has estimated that approximately 12 percent of the American workforce, representing 114 million workers, have alcohol-related problems.[104] The majority of employers surveyed (86%) have stated that alcohol was the number one drug of choice in the workplace regardless of the type of business or industry; e.g., manufacturing, insurance, civil service, transportation, financial services, health care, retailing, education, and others.[105,106] In addition, researchers have indicated that the individual who drinks on the job or abuses alcohol in general is a hazard not only to him/herself but to others as well and that 50 percent of on-the-job problems are alcohol related.[107, 108]

Economic Costs of Alcohol Abuse: It is estimated that approximately $54.7 billion is lost annually in the workplace due to alcohol abuse and alcohol related problems.[109] The estimated economic cost of alcohol abuse and dependence has been determined to be much higher. Harwood and colleagues have projected the cost to steadily increase from $116.9 billion in 1983 to an anticipated $150 billion in 1995.[110] This projected increase is based on the drinking patterns in the United States. Furthermore, approximately $15 billion of the total economic cost is attributed to health care expenditures due to alcohol abuse.

In a review of literature, Holder and Hallan have reported that the average cost of health care for the alcohol abusing or dependent individual is approximately 100 percent higher than for the non-alcohol abusing or dependent employee.[111] As was presented in Chapter 2 of this text, it is not surprising that an alcohol abusing individual may be experiencing either acute or chronic illnesses or traumas as a result of accidents associated with the consequences of alcohol consumption. The secondary complications as a result of alcohol abuse will have a direct effect on the cost of health care.

A. Tardiness and Absenteeism Due to Alcohol-Related Problems

To clearly assess the impact of alcohol abuse on the work environment is difficult, because people who call in sick or late, do not readily admit the cause is alcohol-related. Persons harmfully involved with alcohol or drugs arrive late at work 3 times more frequently than individuals not involved with alcohol or drugs. In addition, individuals with alcohol-related concerns ask for more time off or early dismissals 2.2 times more often than non-alcohol abusing persons.[112]

Individuals abusing alcohol or drugs were absent from work 16 times more frequently than persons not involved with alcohol or drugs. Trice reported that absenteeism appeared to be 3.8 to 8.3 times greater among alcohol abusing individuals than among workers who did not abuse alcohol.[113] Other studies have demonstrated that workers who abuse alcohol were absent 1.5 to 3 times more often than non-alcohol abusing employees.[114] Overall, the rate of absenteeism among alcohol-abusing individuals in the workplace appears to be in the range of 1.5 to 8.3 times greater than for the non-alcohol-abusing worker.

A survey conducted by the EAP Coordinator cited that 74 percent of 53 respondents stated that tardiness and absenteeism was the most significant association between alcohol or drug use and deterioration in work performance.[115]

B. Accidents and Other Consequences of Alcohol Abuse on the Workplace

Sixty-four percent of those surveyed in a study conducted by the EAP Coordinator cited accidents occurred on the job as a result of alcohol abuse. The survey also revealed that 53 percent of those surveyed reported poor quality of work was attributable to alcohol-related reasons as were conflicts with supervisors. Forty-five percent of the respondents cited low quality work and 40 percent reported work not done on time as a consequence of alcohol abuse or dependence.[116]

A study conducted by **Business Month** with 609 executives of companies with revenues in excess of $50 million found that 73 percent saw alcohol and other drug use as a major workplace problem. In addition to absenteeism, tardiness or on the job conflict, the alcohol abusing individual may be involved in accidents three to four times more often than a non-alcohol/drug abusing employee.[117]

The Federal Railway Administration found that drinking problems have cost the railroads $3.1 million in excessive absenteeism, $101 million in lost productivity, $583,000 in injuries, $650,000 in accidental property damage, and $408,000 in grievance procedures.[118]

Consequences of chronic alcohol consumption in the workplace may be especially serious in professions affecting the lives of others. "Catastrophic results may ensue from errors in judgment induced by heavy drinking among, for example, highly placed civil servants, engineers, physicians and surgeons."[119] It is highly important to take into account the fact that regardless of the profession or job setting, if an individual is suspected of an alcohol abuse problem having an impact on his/her job performance, he/she must be identified and referred for help. Whether the individual is an assembly line worker, surgeon, or company supervisor, alcohol-related problems in the workplace have far reaching consequences.

C. Dealing with Alcohol Abuse in the Workplace

In 1971 the Association of Labor-Management Administrators and Consultants on Alcoholism (ALMACA) was set up to look into the critical concerns in the work environment. Today ALMACA is known as the Employee Assistance Professionals Association (EAPA) and among the central concerns of health-care considerations in the workplace is the matter of alcohol abuse. The EAPA is an organization of 6000 individuals directly involved with Employee Assistance Programs (EAPs) nationwide.

The Employee Assistance Programs (EAPs) were set up as a model for intervention and referral of alcohol abusing individuals in the work environment to appropriate in-patient or out-patient alcoholism treatment facilities. Recently, EAPs have determined that the incidence and prevalence of alcohol abuse problems in the workplace comprises between 21 percent and 66 percent of the caseload of employee assistance counselors. It appears that approximately 38 percent of an EAP counselor's workload consists of individuals with alcohol-related problems. At any given time, the caseloads of all EAPs nationally have contact with approximately 600,000 to 1.3 million alcohol-abusing or dependent individuals.[120]

It is estimated that American business and industry employers invest between $204 million and $798 million annually in EAPs. On the upside, however, for every $1 invested in

EAPs, the employers recover from loss an estimated $3 to $5, or an average of $612 million to $3.9 billion annually.[121]

In addition, the Hazeldon Foundation reported that alcohol-related absenteeism dropped from 488 hours before treatment to 168 hours annually after treatment. This figure represents a decline in alcohol-related absenteeism of 66 percent.[122] However, despite the fact that higher health care costs occur in the alcohol-abusing workforce, health care costs do go down after the individual undergoes treatment for alcohol-related problems. It has been shown that the cost to rehabilitate a valuable employee who has alcohol-related problems is more cost-effective than firing and training a new employee. "Treatment is an investment in continued employment of an experienced worker who knows and understands the job and the culture of the work organization."[123]

In conclusion, it is important to look at the human factor affected by alcohol abuse in conjunction with the economic cost to business and industry. Prevention of alcohol abuse in the workplace will be more effective if alcohol abuse and the secondary complications of alcohol consumption are examined and presented to all workers. What may at face value look like acute gastritis complaints may in actuality be an alcohol-related problem. This is not to suggest that every worker complaining of stomach problems, etc. is abusing alcohol. It is merely a recommendation not to exclude or overlook information that will be helpful and necessary for both the worker and the EAP counselor in outlining the most successful course of treatment.

It is evident that treatment for alcoholism with appropriate followup recovery steps is highly effective in returning the individual to work. However, secondary complications (as presented in Chapter 2) must not be overlooked when working with the individual who has a personal or family history of alcohol abuse or dependence.

SUMMARY

Adverse social consequences of alcohol abuse include but are not limited to the following incidents: traffic, aviation, and boating accidents, fires, falls, crime, violence, spouse and child abuse, and problems in the workplace. The key facts pertaining to these social consequences are summarized as follows:

1. Traffic Accidents

Alcohol abuse accounts for approximately two million individuals being arrested each year for drinking and driving. Drunk driving and alcohol related traffic fatalities continue to be one of the Nation's most serious health problems.

2. Aviation

Studies pertaining to alcohol use and flying have revealed that alcohol use decreases motor control and reduces pilot ability to process and integrate information. Alcohol use also can distort equilibrium, and impair coordination and visual-motor skills.

3. Boating Accidents

Alcohol is a significant factor in as many as 65 to 68 percent of all drownings.

4. Fires and Burns

Alcohol consumption has been associated with increased risk of fires and burns. Research has revealed that alcohol abusing individuals were ten times more likely to die because of a fire.

5. Falls

Alcoholics are five to 13 times more likely to die from falls as compared with non-alcohol abusing individuals.

6. Traumatic Injuries

Two of the most serious injuries sustained because of alcohol intoxication are traumatic brain injury and spinal cord injury. Alcohol is the strongest predisposing element in traumatic brain injury and 50 percent of all traumatic brian injury is alcohol-related. 68 percent of all disabling spinal cord injuries are the result of alcohol and/or drug use at the time of injury.

7. Crime and Violence

Individuals who engage in criminal activity are more likely to have alcohol abuse problems. It has been documented that the higher the level of intoxication, the greater the severity and number of injuries sustained in assaultive or violent behavior. Excessive alcohol consumption in the family has been associated with various degrees of emotional and physical abuse. Alcohol has been cited in 45 to 60 percent of all cases of spouse abuse and 17 percent of all reported cases of child abuse. Additionally, the result of spouse or child abuse quite often is manifested in post-traumatic stress disorder.

8. Work Environment

Approximately 12 percent or 14 million workers in the U.S. have alcohol-related problems. Moreover, fifty percent of all on-the-job problems are alcohol related. The alcohol abusing person is 3 to 4 times more likely to be involved in an on-the-job accident than a non alcohol-abusing employee.

With the voluminous documentation of how alcohol abuse impacts on society together with the various debilitating consequences of such abuse (e.g. traumatic brain injury, spinal cord injury, post-traumatic stress disorder, etc.), it is critical that counselors address alcohol use and abuse issues with all survivors and victims of alcohol-related accidents and violence.

Alcohol counseling must be a component of all rehabilitation services dealing with the traumatic aftermath of alcohol-related incidents in order to prevent the onset of alcohol abusing behaviors or recidivism of existing alcoholism.

REFERENCES

1. Department of Health and Human Services DHHS), **Fifth Special Report to the U. S. Congress on Alcohol and Health**, DHHS #ADM 84-1291, USGPO, Washington, D. C. 1983.
2. National Highway Traffic Safety Administration, **Fact Sheet on Alcohol-Impaired Driving**, DHHS #MS384, National Clearinghouse for Alcohol and Drug Information, Rockville, Maryland, 1988.
3. National Highway Traffic Safety Administration, **Drunk Driving Facts**, #RPO717, National Center for Statistics and Analysis, Washington, D. C., July 1989.
4. National Highway Traffic Safety Administration, **Alcohol Involvement in Fatal Crashes**, Rep. #DOT HS 807, NHTSA, Washington, D. C., 1988.
5. National Highway Traffic Safety Administration, **Drunk**, 1989.
6. National Highway Traffic Safety Administration, **National Accident Sampling System 1986**, NHTSA, Washington, D. C., 1988.
7. Meyers, H. B., Zepeda, S. G., and Murdock, M. A., Alcohol and trauma: An endemic syndrome, **The Western Journal of Medicine, 153**, 149-154, 1990.
8. National Highway Traffic Safety Administration, **Drunk**, 1989.

9. Fell, J. C., Drinking and driving in America: Disturbing facts - encouraging reductions, **Alcohol Health and Research World, 14,** 18-26, 1990.

10. CDC: Youth drinking-related crash deaths down, **Alcoholism and Drug Abuse Week, 3,** 5, March 27, 1991.

11. Oei, T. P. S. and Kerschbaumer, D. M., Peer attitudes, sex, and the effect of alcohol on simulated driving performance, **American Journal of Drug and Alcohol Abuse, 16,** 135-146, 1990.

12. Vegega, M. E. and Klein, T. M., Alcohol-related traffic fatalities among youth and young adults - United States, 1982-1989, **The Journal of the American Medical Association, 165,** 1930-1931, April 17, 1991.

13. Novelle, A., Teen drinking habits alarm Surgeon General, **Alcoholism ad Drug Abuse Week, 3,** 4, 1991.

14. Ross, L. E. and Ross, S. M., Alcohol and drug use in aviation, **Alcohol Health and Research World, 9**(4), 34-41, 1985.

15. Modell, J. G. and Mountz, J. M., Drinking and flying - the problem of alcohol use by pilots, **The New England Journal of Medicine, 323,** 455-462, August 16, 1990.

16. Effects of alcohol on pilot performance in simulated flight, **The Journal of the American Medical Association, 265,** 2796, June 5, 1991.

17. Modell, **Drinking,** 1990.

18. Porterfield, K. M., And the loser is. . . the drinking athlete, **Current Health, 17,** 18-20, October 2, 1990.

19. Ross, **Alcohol,** 1985.

20. Baker, S. P., O'Neil, B., and Karpf, R., **Injury Fact Book,** Heath, Lexington, Massachusetts, 1984.

21. Alcohol use and aquatic activities - Massachusetts, **The Journal of the American Medical Association, 264,** 19-21, July 4, 1990.

22. Wright, S. J., SOS: Alcohol, drugs and boating, **Alcohol Health and Research World, 9**(4), 28-33, 1985.

23. Bernhartsen, J., I never saw the other boat, **Countermeasure, 5,** 7, 1984.

24. Wright, SOS, 1985.

25. National Transportation Safety Board, **Safety Study: Recreational Boating Safety and Alcohol**, NTSB, Washington, D. C., 1983.

26. Stanley, R. J. and Siegal, G. P., **Death by drowning: An overview, Minnesota Medicine, 64**(5), 295-297, 1981.

27. **Alcohol use**, 1990.

28. Baker, **Injury**, 1984.

29. Department of Health and Human Services, **Seventh**, 1990.

30. Waller, J. A., Nonhighway injury fatalities - The roles of alcohol and problem drinking, drugs and medical impairment, **Journal of Chronic Diseases, 25,** 33-45, 1972.

31. Howland, J. and Hingson, R., Alcohol as a risk factor for injuries or death due to fires and burns: Review of the literature, **Public Health Report, 102,** 475-483, 1987.

32. National Safety Council, **Accident Facts 1984**, National Safety Council, Chicago, Illinois, 1984.

33. Schmidt, W. and DeLint J., Cause of death of alcoholics, **Quarterly Journal of Studies on Alcohol, 33,** 171-185, 1972.

34. Baker, **Injury**, 1984.

35. Department of Health and Human Services, **Seventh**, 1990.

36. Nicholls, P., Edwards, G., and Kyle, E., Alcoholics admitted to four hospitals in England: General and cause specific mortality, **Quarterly Journal of Studies on Alcohol, 33,** 841-855, 1974.

37. Schmidt, W. and De Lint, J., Cause of death of alcoholics, **Quarterly Journal of Studies on Alcohol, 33,** 171-185, 1972.

38. Podolsky, D. M., The not-so-safe refuge: Unintentional injuries in the home and

at play, **Alcohol Health and Research World,** **9**(4), 24-27, 1985.

39. Honkanen, R., Ertama, L., Kuosmanen, P., Linnoila, M., Alha, A., and Visuri, T., The role of alcohol in accidental falls, **Journal of Studies on Alcohol, 44,** 231-245, 1983.

40. Field, J. H., **Epidemiology of Head Injury in England and Wales: With Particular Application to Rehabilitation,** Willsons, Leicester, England, 1976.

41. Jones, G. A., Alcohol abuse and traumatic brain injury, **Alcohol Health and Research World, 13,** 104-109, 1989.

42. Parkinson, D., Stephenson, S., and Phillips S., Head injuries: A prospective, computerized study, **Canadian Journal of Surgery, 28**(1), 79-83, 1985.

43. Slaby, A. E., Lieb, J., and Tancredi, L. R., **Handbook of Psychiatric Emergencies,** 2nd Ed., Medical Examination Publishing, Garden City, New York, 1981.

44. After the fall, **Harvard Health Letter, 16**(6), 1-3, April 1991.

45. Jones, **Alcohol,** 1989.

46. Jones, **Alcohol,** 1989.

47. Alterman, A. I., Tarter, R. E., Relationship between familial alcoholism and head injury, **Journal of Studies on Alcohol, 46**(3), 256-258, 1985.

48. **After the fall,** 1991.

49. Jones, **Alcohol,** 1989.

50. Mitiguy, J., **Alcohol and head trauma, Headlines, 2**(2), 2, 1991.

51. Sparadeo, F. and Gill, D., Effects of prior alcohol use on head injury recovery, **Journal Head Trauma Rehabilitation, 4**(1), 75-82, 1989.

52. Mitiguy, **Alcohol,** 1991.

53. Wasco, J., Attacking the problem before it starts, **Headlines, 2**(2), 20, 1991.

54. Kaitz, S., Integrated treatment: Safety net for survival, **Headlines, 2**(2), 10, 1991.

55. Mitiguy, **Alcohol,** 1991.

56. Sparadeo, **Effects**, 1989.

57. Reilly, E. L., Kelley, J. T., and Faillace, L. A., Role of alcohol use and abuse in trauma, **Advances in Psychosomatic Medicine, 16**, 17-30, 1986.

58. Kaitz, **Integrated**, 1991.

59. Kelly, A., Spinal cord injury: Facts, figures, rehab., **Independent Living, 6**, 47-49, 1991.

60. O'Donnell, J. J., Cooper, J. E., Gessner, J. E., Shehan, I., and Ashley, J., Alcohol, drugs and spinal cord injury, **Alcohol Health and Research World, 6**, 27-29, 1981-82.

61. Heinemann, A. W., Doll, M., and Schnoll, S., Treatment of alcohol abuse in persons with recent spinal cord injuries, **Alcohol Health and Research World, 13**(2), 110-117, 1989.

62. Heinemann, A., Donohue, R., Keen, M., and Schnoll, S., Alcohol use by persons with recent spinal cord injuries, **Archives of Physical Medicine and Rehabilitation, 69**, 619-624, 1988.

63. Rasmussen, G. and DeBoer, R., Alcohol and drug use among clients at a residential vocational rehabilitation facility, **Alcohol Health and Research World, 5**, 48-56, 1980-81.

64. Heinemann, **Treatment**, 1989.

65. Dufour, M. C., Bertolucci, D., Cowell, C., Stinson, F. S., and Noble, J., Alcohol-related morbidity among the disabled, **Alcohol Health and Research World, 13**(2), 158-161, 1989.

66. Schaschl, S. and Straw, D., Results of a model intervention program for physically impaired persons, **Alcohol Health and Research World, 13**(2), 150-153, 1989.

67. Room, R., Alcohol and crime: Behavioral aspects, in **Encyclopedia of Crime and Justice**, Vol. 1, 35-44, Kadish, S. H., Ed., Free Press, New York, 1983.

68. Siann, G., **Accounting for Aggression: Perspectives on Aggression and Violence**, Allen and Unwin, Boston, 1985.

69. Alcohol and violence (editorial), **The Lancet, 336**, 1223-1225, November 17, 1990.
70. NIAAA, **Medical**, 1984.
71. Greenberg, S. W., Alcohol and crime: A methodologic critique of the literature, in Drinking and Crime: **Perspectives on the Relationships Between Alcohol Consumption and Criminal Behavior**, 70-109, Collins, J. J., Ed., Guilford Press, New York, 1981.
72. Baunach, P., Jail inmates, **Bureau of Justice Statistics Bulletin**, Rep. #NCJ-99175, U. S. Department of Justice, Washington, D. C., 1983.
73. NIAAA, **Medical**, 1984.
74. Loberg, R., Belligerence in alcohol dependence, **Scandinavian Journal of Psychology, 24**, 285-292, 1983.
75. Pihl, R., Alcohol and aggression: A psychological perspective, in **Alcohol, Drug Abuse and Aggression**, 292-313, Gottheil, E., Druley, K. A., Skoloda, T. E., Waxman, H. M., Eds., Charles Thomas, Springfield, Connecticut, 1983.
76. Jensen, R., Severity of delinquent offenses and alcohol involvement among residents in a Midwestern correctional facility, **Juvenile and Family Court Journal, 33**(4), 63-66, 1982.
77. Dawkins, M. P. and Dawkins, R. L., Alcohol use and delinquency among black, white and Hispanic adolescent offenders, **Adolescence, 18**(72), 799-809, 1983.
78. Lystad, M., **Violence in the Home: Interdisciplinary Perspectives**, Brunner/Mazel, New York, 1986.
79. Hindman, M. H., Family violence: An overview, **Alcohol Health and Research World, 4**(1), 2-11, 1979.
80. Roy, M., A research project probing a cross-section of battered women: A current survey of 150 cases, in **Battered Women: A Psychological Study of Domestic Violence**, 225-244, Roy, M., Ed., Van Nostrand, New York, 1977.

81. Flanzer, J., Alcohol abuse and family violence: The domestic chemical connection, **Family Focus and Chemical Dependency, 7**(4), 5-6, 1984.

82. Roy, **Research**, 1977.

83. Paolino, R. J. and McCrady, B. S., **The Alcoholic Marriage: Alternative Perspectives**, Grune and Stratton, New York, 1977.

84. Jacob, R. and Seilhamer, R., The impact on spouses and how they cope, in **Alcohol and the Family**, 114-126, Orford, J. and Harwin, J., Eds., St. Martin's Press, New York, 1982.

85. Hamilton, C. J. and Collins, J. J., Jr., The role of alcohol in wife beating and child abuse: A review of the literature, in **Drinking and Crime: Perspective on the Relationships between Alcohol Consumption and Criminal Behavior**, 253-287, Collins, J. J., Jr., Ed., Guilford Press, New York, 1981.

86. Hamilton, **Role**, 1981.

87. Kantor, G. K. and Straus, M. A., The "drunken burn" theory of wife beating, **Social Problems, 34**(3), 214-230, 1987.

88. Bland, R. and Orn, H., Family violence and psychiatric disorder, **Canadian Journal of Psychiatry, 31**, 129-137, 1986.

89. Van Hasselt, V., Morrison, R., and Bellack, A., Alcohol use in wife abusers and their spouses, **Addictive Behavior, 10**, 127-135, 1985.

90. Department of Health and Human Services (DHHS), **Fifth Special Report to the U. S. Congress on Alcohol and Health**, DHHS Rep. #ADM 84-1291, USGPO, Washington, D. C., 1983.

91. Bland, **Family**, 1986.

92. Chafetz, M., Blane, H., and Hill, M., Children of alcoholics, **Quarterly Journal of Studies on Alcohol, 32**, 687-698, 1971.

93. Christopoulos, C., Cohn, D. A., Shaw, D. S., Joyce, S., Sullivan-Hanson, J., Kraft, S., and Emery, R. E., Children of abused women: I. Adjustment at time of shelter residence, **Journal of Marriage and the Family, 49**, 611-619, 1987.

94. Rosenberg, M. S., New directions for research on the psychological maltreatment of children, **American Psychologist, 42**, 166-171.

95. Cummings, E. M., Coping with background anger in early childhood, **Child Development, 58**, 976-984, 1987.

96. Emery, R. E., Interparental conflict and the children of discord and divorce, **Psychological Bulletin, 92**, 310-330, 1982.

97. Figley, C. R., Catastrophes: An overview of family reactions, in **Stress and the Family**, 3-20, Figley, C. R. and McCubbin, H. I., Eds., Brunner/Mazel, New York, 1983.

98. Lifton, R. J., **The Broken Connection**, Simon and Schuster, New York, 1979.

99. Frederick, C., Effects of natural versus human-induced violence upon the victim, **Evaluation and Change**, 71-75, 1980.

100. Putnam, R. W., Post, R. M., and Guroff, J. J., One hundred cases of multiple personality disorder. Presented at the annual meeting of the American Psychiatric Association, Los Angeles, California, May 1984.

101. American Psychiatric Association, **Diagnostic and Statistical Manual**, 3rd Ed., Revised, (**DSM-III-R**) American Psychiatric Press, Washington, D. C., 1987.

102. Robertson, B. E., **Life Experiences of Adult Daughters of Alcoholics: A Qualitative Study**, UMI, Ann Arbor, Michigan, 1989.

103. Marge, M., The prevention of human disabilities: Policies and practices for the 80s, in **International Aspects of Rehabilitation of Disabled Persons: Policy Guidance for the 1980s**, 11-22, Perlman, L. G., Ed., National Rehabilitation Association, Alexandria, Virginia, 1980.

104. Employee Assistance Professionals Association (EAPA), **Facts About Employer Investment in Employees Assistance Programs**, EAPA, Arlington, Virginia, June 6, 1989.

105. Employee Assistance Professionals Association, **Four Most Prevalent Workplace Drugs**, EAPA, Arlington, Virginia, May 19, 1989.
106. Employee Assistance Professionals Association, **Facts About the Incidence and Prevalence of Alcohol Abuse/Other Drug Use and Other Life Problems in the Workplace**, EAPA, Arlington, Virginia, May 10, 1989.
107. Chafetz, **Children**, 1971.
108. NIAAA, **Medical** 1984.
109. EAPA, **Facts About Employer**, 1989.
110. Harwood, H. J., Kristiansen, P., and Rachal, J. V., **Social and Economic Costs of Alcohol Abuse and Alcoholism**. Rep. #2, Research Triangle Institute, Research Triangle Park, North Carolina, 1985.
111. Holder, H. D. and Hallan, J. B., Impact of alcoholism treatment on total health care costs: A six-year study, **Advances in Alcohol and Substance Abuse,** 6(1), 1-15, 1986.
112. Employee Assistance Professionals Association, **Facts About Absenteeism**, EAPA, Arlington, Virginia, May 22, 1989.
113. Trice, H., Job based alcoholism and employee assistance programs, **Alcohol Health and Research World,** 4(3), 4, 1980.
114. EAPA, **Facts About Absenteeism**, 1989.
115. EAPA, **Facts About Impact**, 1989.
116. EAPA, **Facts About Impact**, 1989.
117. EAPA, **Facts About Impact**, 1989.
118. EAPA, **Facts About Impact**, 1989.
119. Moser, J., **Prevention of Alcohol-Related Problems: An International Review of Preventive Measures, Policies and Programmes**, Alcoholism and Drug Addiction Research Foundation, Toronto, Canada, 1980.
120. EAPA, **Facts About Impact**, 1989.
121. Employee Assistance Professionals Association, **Facts About Employer Investment in Employee Assistance Programs**, EAPA, Arlington, Virginia, June 6, 1989.
122. EAPA, **Four**, 1989.
123. Employee Assistance Professionals

Association, **Facts About Termination Versus Treatment**, EAPA, Arlington, Virginia, May 10, 1989.

Chapter 4

ALCOHOLISM, DRUGS AND TOBACCO

I. ALCOHOLISM

Alcoholism is not only one of the causes of human disabilities, it is also considered one of the most prevalent disabilities in and of itself in the United States. How prevalent is the use of alcohol in the United States to be concerned about alcoholism being both a disability and the cause of a number of preventable disabilities? In the United States in the late eighties, 5.8 billion gallons of beer, 583.3 million gallons of wine, and 394.7 million gallons of spirits were sold. Averaging these figures to include each person in the United States aged 14 years and older, the previous amounts would represent the following - 291.8 gallons of beer, 3 gallons of wine, and 2.1 gallons of spirits consumed per person annually.[1] Taking into consideration that approximately one-third of the population does not consume alcoholic beverages, the figures presented are an underestimate of the actual annual consumption of alcoholic beverages per person who does drink alcohol.

Measuring the prevalence of alcohol consumption in society is highly important since the extent of the problem can be measured by the amount of alcohol consumed. In other words, the more alcohol consumed, the greater the likelihood of alcohol-related problems. Based on the high numbers of alcohol use, it is evident that the consumption of alcoholic beverages may significantly contribute to the causes and/or the course and outcome of a number of physical, behavioral, and psychosocial problems.[2]

More often than not, when a person sees a physician for a physical complaint, he or she may be diagnosed on the basis of the secondary complications that have resulted as a consequence of acute or chronic alcohol abuse or dependence. The person finds him/herself receiving medical care for the secondary complications or symptoms of alcoholism rather than for the cause of the symptoms and physical complaints - alcohol abuse or dependence. Upon closer scrutiny, the primary diagnosis in many cases may be alcoholism rather than, for example, gastritis. Gastritis in this case would be a co-existing diagnosis. One of the reasons for not addressing alcoholism as a primary problem on the part of the physician may be due to the fact that many physicians indicate that they do not know enough about alcohol or other drug problems.[3] However, treating a physical ailment without taking into account alcoholism will only lead to dire consequences for the individual.

Alcoholism can be an individual's only disability or it can be a precursor to or occur with other debilitating physical or psychiatric disabilities.[4] When alcoholism is diagnosed as the person's only disability, it is due to the fact that no physical or psychiatric complications have ensued as a result of alcohol abuse or dependence. However, alcoholism may have complicated the individual's life in the workplace, the family, financially, legally (e.g., DWI), or socially. In this case, the individual diagnosed with alcohol abuse or dependence must seek treatment for the primary disability of alcoholism.

The National Council on Alcoholism (NCA) and the American Medical Society on Alcoholism (AMSA) have defined alcoholism as a chronic, progressive and potentially fatal disease.[5, 6] Not only is alcoholism a chronic and progressive disease, it is also incurable. As long as the person drinks, the person is on a downward spiral toward a debilitating disability or death. Alcoholism is also characterized by loss of control over alcohol and over other sedative drugs (e.g., tranquilizers, sleeping pills). In other words, one drink leads to the next and so on.

Although the debate continues as to whether alcoholism is a disease or not, most practitioners in the field of alcohol and substance abuse do accept the disease concept. For alcoholism to be accepted as a disease as scientific fact rather than theory or conjecture, the following criteria for a disease must be met. All diseases have a cause (either known or idiopathic), symptoms, signs or physical findings, pathogenesis or course of illness, outcome, and treatment. Jellinek is credited with formulating the theory that alcoholism was a disease with predictable signs and symptoms.[7] In addition, Jellinek found that many alcoholics go through a series of stages from relatively harmless consequences of drinking to very serious and debilitating or fatal results. The downward course of alcoholism based on Jellinek's concept of alcoholism as a disease and illustrated by Ohlms is as follows:

A. STAGES OF DRINKING
1. Early Stage of Drinking
- Drinking alcohol for relief from emotional pain or stress
- Blackouts or periods of memory loss
- Driving while intoxicated
- Loss of control over drinking

2. Middle Stage of Drinking
- Marital and family problems due to drinking
- Problems on the job as a result of drinking
- Financial problems as a result of drinking
- Legal problems incurred (e.g., arrested for DWI)
- Changes in personality or behavior

3. **Late Stage of Drinking**
   - Secondary physical and/or mental complications
   - Death

Unless a person seeks helps for alcoholism during the early or middle stages of alcoholism, the progression toward secondary complications as seen in the late stage of drinking is inevitable. In many cases an individual is not even considered an alcoholic until he or she is in the late stage of drinking.[9] Unfortunately, when a person reaches the late stage of drinking and physical or mental deterioration has developed, oftentimes there is damage that could have been arrested or prevented had the person been referred for treatment earlier.

Nowadays, individuals are referred for treatment for alcohol abuse or dependence based on history of DWIs (e.g., number of DWIs, BAC levels). With referral for treatment during the early or middle stages of drinking, it is hopeful that physical damage may be prevented and psychosocial problems be averted. But despite what is known today regarding the severe problems that chronic alcohol consumption can cause, 96 percent of alcoholics still die due to either secondary complications or as a result of traumatic and violent accidents (e.g., car crashes, falls, etc.) suffered while under the influence of alcohol. However, if treatment is sought for alcohol abuse or dependence, seventy to eighty percent of alcoholics will recover.[10]

When an individual seeks treatment for alcohol abuse or dependence, he or she must meet certain criteria for alcoholism to be considered a primary diagnosis. The **DSM-III-R** has established the following diagnostic criteria for psychoactive substance abuse in which alcohol is one of the nine classes of psychoactive substances associated with both abuse and dependence:

Psychoactive Substance <u>Dependence</u> (Alcohol):
a. At least three of the following:
   (1) substance often taken in larger amounts or over a longer period than the person intended,
   (2) persistent desire or one or more unsuccessful efforts to cut down or control substance use.
   (3) a great deal of time spent in activities necessary to get the substance, or recovering from its effects,
   (4) frequent intoxication or withdrawal symptoms when expected to fulfill major role obligations at work, school, or home (e.g., does not go to work because hung over, goes to school or work "high", intoxicated while taking care of his or her children, or when substance use is physically hazardous (e.g., drives when intoxicated),
   (5) important social, occupational, or recreational activities given up or reduced because of substance use,
   (6) continued substance use despite knowledge of having a persistent or recurrent social, psychological, or physical problem that is caused or exacerbated by the use of the substance (e.g., ulcer made worse by drinking),
   (7) marked tolerance: need for markedly increased amounts of the substance (i.e., at least a 50 percent increase) in order to achieve intoxication or desired effect, or markedly diminished effect with continued use of the same amount,
   (8) characteristic withdrawal symptoms,
   (9) substance often taken to relieve or avoid withdrawal symptoms.
b. Some symptoms of the disturbance have persisted for at least one month, or have occurred repeatedly over a longer period of time.

Psychoactive Substance Abuse (Alcohol):
a. A maladaptive pattern of psychoactive substance use indicated by at least one of the following:
(1) continued use despite knowledge of having a persistent or recurrent social, occupational, psychological, or physical problem that is caused or exacerbated by use of the psychoactive substance,
(2) recurrent use in situations in which use is physically hazardous (e.g., driving while intoxicated).
b. Some symptoms of the disturbance have persisted for at least one month, or have occurred repeatedly over a longer period of time.
c. Never met the criteria for psychoactive substance dependence for this substance.

Once the person meets the criteria for either alcohol abuse or alcohol dependence, the treatment plan is set according to severity and chronicity of problem. The treatment plan may consist of either out-patient or inpatient treatment.

II. DRUG ABUSE

Researchers have reported that drug abuse on the part of alcoholics is a frequent occurrence. In a review of 44 studies investigating drug abuse among alcoholics, Grande and colleagues found an 80 percent connection between alcoholism and drug abuse.[12] Other studies revealed a prevalence rate of drug abuse among alcoholics between 20 percent and 80 percent.[13] In 1985, the combined use of alcohol and any other drug accounted for 66.3 percent of all drug-related episodes reported by emergency rooms.[14] Furthermore, reports have revealed that one-third of all individuals who use alcohol also use other drugs, and two-thirds of drug abusers also use alcohol.[15] A report from the National

Institute on Drug Abuse revealed that problems associated with the use of drugs often include the accompanying use of alcohol.[16]

Drugs of choice among alcoholics vary according to age.[17] Whereas older alcoholics abuse prescription drugs such as tranquilizers and other sedative-hypnotics, younger alcoholics abuse amphetamines, marijuana, cocaine and other illicit drugs. It is not surprising that older alcoholics abuse sedative-hypnotics since an increased tolerance to alcohol (due to long term alcohol consumption) will produce the same desired effect by most sedative-hypnotics. This increased tolerance to sedative-hypnotics based on an increased tolerance to alcohol is called cross-tolerance.

The main reason for cross-tolerance between alcohol and sedative-hypnotic drugs is the fact that alcohol falls into the same pharmacological category. Alcohol, barbiturates (e.g., Nembutal, Seconal, etc.), benzodiazepines (e.g., Valium, Librium, etc.), anesthetics, and antihistamines are central nervous system depressants or "downers", and all are classified as sedative-hypnotics.[18] But despite the fact that alcohol and other sedative hypnotics fall into the same class, using alcohol together with another sedative-hypnotic drug does not double the effect of the two substances. The effect becomes greater than the sum total of the individual effects. This increased effect is called synergism.

Synergistic interactions often produce unexpected and dangerous interactions. For example, combining alcohol with a barbiturate (e.g., Seconal) may result in a severely depressed central nervous system. Rather than experiencing deep relaxation and sleep, the alcoholic may find him or herself in a coma.[19] Even a small amount of alcohol combined with any other sedative-hypnotic can result in an accident or death because of the unexpected synergistic effect.

However, individuals who abuse alcohol and drugs do not always seek the same effects from one drug or substance that they derive from another. On the contrary, many substance abusers will use one drug to counteract the undesired effects of another. For example, the use of alcohol may be used to offset the excessive stimulation derived from cocaine use. The combined use of alcohol and cocaine was reported as one of the most dangerous combinations and has resulted in the largest number of emergency episodes or drug-related deaths. The dangerous combination of alcohol and heroin was reported as the second cause of polydrug-related emergencies and deaths reported by medical examiners.[20] Clinicians also found that alcohol was the most common substance abused by cocaine users.[21] Across both genders, cocaine and heroin were the drugs most frequently used with alcohol.[22] Overall, the National Institute on Drug Abuse reported the drugs that were used the most extensively with alcohol were cocaine, Valium, heroin, morphine, and phencyclidine (PCP).

Combining alcohol with another drug increases the possibility that the individual may encounter or cause an injury, disability, or death. Several studies have identified the fact that combining alcohol with another drug is a significant factor in motor vehicle accidents that result in severe injury or death, and in criminal activity.[23,24]

In regard to adolescent or young adult use of alcohol and drugs, it was reported that alcohol consumption was a prerequisite to the use of marijuana, psychedelics, amphetamines, barbiturates, cocaine, and heroin.[25] Despite the emphasis on drug abuse among youth, alcohol still remains the most available and widespread of substances of abuse among the young. An estimated 4.6 million adolescents or one-third of all 14 to 17 year olds have a serious problem with alcohol.[26]

Johnston, O'Malley and Bachman reported that 92 percent of all high school seniors surveyed in the National High School Senior Survey had tried alcohol and 66 percent were active users of alcohol. In addition, 57 percent of high school seniors reported having tried an illicit drug and 36 percent reported using an illicit drug other than marijuana. Cocaine was tried by 15.2 percent of all high school seniors and 5.6 percent had tried crack.[27]

Among the reasons for the high percentage of alcohol users among high school youth is the fact that alcohol is easily accessible, it is low in cost, and, generally, socially acceptable.[28] Although alcohol may be socially acceptable, behaviors resulting from alcohol and drug use are not. There is an increase in delinquent and antisocial behaviors among adolescents and young adults that use and abuse alcohol and/or drugs. Hawkins, Lishner, Jenson & Catalano reported that frequent use and abuse of alcohol and drugs is more common among youth who commit crimes or engage in delinquent behavior.[29] Elliott & Huizinga reported that alcohol use among delinquents was 4 to 9 times higher than among nonoffenders.[30] In a study conducted with juvenile offenders sentenced for a violent crime, 50 percent reported using alcohol and/or drugs prior to the violent activity. Furthermore, it was found that approximately two to six percent of all youth continue the frequent use of alcohol and drugs and criminal activity into their adult life.[31]

In addition to the consequences of antisocial behavior as a result of alcohol and/or drug abuse, the young person is also vulnerable to the myriad of secondary complications (physical and psychiatric, discussed in Chapter 2 of this text). A note of caution: although alcohol and/or drug abuse on the part of the adolescent or young adult may lead to delinquent or criminal activity, it does not suggest that alcohol and/or drug use causes such behaviors. Another disturbing finding of alcohol and drug use is among individuals who are physically impaired as a consequence of alcohol and/or drug use and continue to combine the use of alcohol with either prescription medications or other drugs. In a study conducted with orthopedically impaired college students, it was reported that orthopedically impaired individuals may be more vulnerable to abusing alcohol and other drugs. This increased vulnerability to abuse both alcohol and drugs may be due to the availability of alcohol in combination with the medication prescribed to ameliorate pain. At the same time antidepressants may be prescribed to relieve depression experienced by the disabled individual due to loss of mobility, low self-esteem, anger, or social isolation. However, after conducting a study with 57 orthopedically impaired college students, Moore and Siegel found that the use of alcohol and drugs among these students correlated most highly with social and euphoriant effects, rather than seeking stress or pain reduction. In this respect the orthopedically impaired students were no different than other college students in the reasons behind the use of alcohol and drugs.[32]

These findings, however, are disturbing in that 61.4 percent of these students reported the use of at least one prescribed drug, 48.7 percent reported using at least three prescribed medications, and 14.3 percent reported using at least five prescribed drugs.[33] Knowing the unpredictable synergistic effects of combining alcohol with sedative-hypnotics, or the dangerous effects of using alcohol and drugs that counteract each other, the danger of injury, accident, or death is an underlying factor in continuing this activity. Unfortunately, many practitioners tend to overlook the use and abuse of alcohol and other drugs among the physically disabled population and focus on the primary physical disability.

In view of the fact that trauma-related disabilities are often correlated with alcohol and drug use at time of injury, it is imperative that practitioners working with the disabled take into consideration the individual's pre-disability and current drinking and drug using activity. Successful rehabilitation and prevention of further injury or death can only result if alcohol and drug history is taken into account and dealt with openly.

III. TOBACCO

Individuals that consume alcohol smoke cigarettes at a considerably higher rate than nondrinkers.[34] It appears that alcohol and tobacco consumption are highly correlated.[35] In a study conducted of very addictive drugs, researchers found that between 80 and 95 percent of individuals who undergo treatment for alcoholism were also cigarette smokers.[36] Drinkers smoke more than nondrinkers and smokers consume more alcohol than do nonsmokers. One study showed that as smoking increased, so did alcohol consumption.[37] In a review of literature, McCoy & Napier indicated that research studies in the last 30 years have shown that the incidence of and mortality from cancers of the head and neck have significantly increased in males who were both heavy smokers and drinkers.[38]

Among women, it was found that maternal alcoholism was often accompanied by smoking and heavy caffeine consumption.[39] In a study of 1117 pregnant women attending an antenatal clinic, researchers observed that the incidence of smoking increased among women who were heavier drinkers.[40] Chapter 1 presents in detail how alcohol consumption significantly contributes to Fetal Alcohol

Syndrome. However, in addition to alcohol use and abuse among pregnant women, smoking was also identified as a high risk factor in contributing to fetal complications and/or abnormalities. Although alcohol and cigarette smoking independently contribute to intrauterine growth retardation (IUGR), the combined use of alcohol and tobacco was found to increase the risk factor of IUGR from a twofold to fourfold incidence.[41-44]

The synergistic effect identified in combining alcohol with sedative-hypnotics has also been identified with smoking and alcohol consumption. In fact, the synergistic effect of smoking and drinking was found to be especially dangerous.[45] Numerous studies have reported that the risks associated with drinking and smoking multiply when the use of alcohol and tobacco is simultaneous.

This synergy or "multiplicative hypothesis" was evidenced in a study of smokers and drinkers who were diagnosed with laryngeal cancer.[46] In this investigation of the joint effects of using alcohol and tobacco simultaneously, the researchers concluded that the relative risks of developing laryngeal cancer among heavy drinkers who also smoke was dramatically increased. Rothman, Cann and Fried also found that there was an increased risk pattern among smokers who drank dark liquor in developing hypopharyngeal cancer.[47]

In addition to laryngeal and hypopharyngeal cancers, researchers concluded that smoking and alcohol consumption were the strongest risk factors for oral cancer and cancer of the tongue. In fact, researchers estimated that the combined effect of heavy drinking and smoking increased the risk of oral cancer more than 15 times as compared with those individuals who neither smoked nor drank.[48,49] It was found that the combined effects of smoking and drinking supported the multiplicative model or the synergistic effect of simultaneously smoking and drinking beverage alcohol.[50,51] Researchers have reported that as many as 75 percent of cancers of the mouth, oropharynx and larynx reported by the National Cancer Institute in 1982 were the result of the combined effects of chronic alcohol and tobacco use.[52]

In general, studies conducted worldwide (e.g., Uruguay, England, China, Germany, United States, and Russia) on the effects of smoking and drinking have concluded that a synergistic or multiplicative effect exists when tobacco and alcohol were used simultaneously. The multiplicative effect rather than merely additive effect of smoking and drinking greatly increases the risk of various cancers, fetal complications and/or abnormalities, and secondary physical complications.

SUMMARY

Although alcoholism is one of the most debilitating disabilities in the U.S., all too often it is the secondary physical or psychiatric complication that is treated. Not addressing alcoholism as a bona fide disability, presents dire consequences for the individual. The "band aid" approach to treating symptoms rather than causes of diseases or illnesses caused by alcohol abuse sends the individual on a downward spiral of ill health and eventual death.

Moreover, the connection between alcohol, drugs and tobacco has been well documented. Research has shown dramatic evidence that alcohol use and abuse is a frequent occurrence among users of both prescription and illegal drugs. There is also a strong correlation between tobacco use and alcoholism. The hazard that exists with the combined use of alcohol and tobacco is the synergistic or multiplicative effect that greatly increases the risk of various diseases or physical complications.

The National Council on Alcoholism and Drug Dependence and the American Medical Society have defined alcoholism as a chronic, progressive and potentially fatal disease. Alcohol abuse must be addressed in the early stages of the disease. Treating the physical and psychiatric complications of alcohol abuse in the late stage benefits no one and the disease or illness that was once preventable becomes irreversible or fatal.

REFERENCES

1. Ethanol consumption in the United States, **Nutrition Research Newsletter, 9**, 33, March 1990.
2. Ashley, M. J., How extensive is the problem of alcoholism? **Alcohol Health and Research World, 13**, 305, 1989.
3. Arkin, E. B. and Funkhouser, J. E., Eds. **Communicating About Alcohol and Other Drugs: Strategies for Reaching Populations at Risk**, Office for Substance Abuse Prevention, Rockville, Maryland, 1990.
4. Fox, V., Conway, J. P., and Schweigler, J., Alcoholism, in **Handbook of Severe Disabilities**, Clowers, S., Ed., U. S. Government Printing Office, 1982, Chap. 17.
5. National Council on Alcoholism (NCA), Criteria for the diagnosing of alcoholism, **American Journal of Psychiatry, 192**, 127, 1972.
6. National Council on Alcoholism and Drug Dependence (NCADD), **Definition of Alcoholism**, NCADD, New York, 1990.
7. Jellinek, E. M., **The Disease Concept of Alcoholism**, College and University Press, New Haven, Connecticut, 1960.
8. Ohlms, D., **Disease Concept of Alcholism, Part II**, (Video), Gary Whiteaker Company, 1984.

9. Ohlms, **Disease**, 1984.
10. Ohlms, **Disease**, 1984.
11. American Psychiatric Association, **Diagnostic and Statistical Manual**, 3rd Ed. revised,(**DSM-III-R**) American Psychiatric Press, Washington, D. C., 1987.
12. Grande, T. P., Wolfe, A. W., Schubert, D. S. P., Patterson, M. B., and Brocco, K., Associations among alcoholism, drug abuse, and anti-social personality; A review of the literature, **Psychological Reports, 55,** 455, 1984.
13. Malloy, T. E., Toward a generic concept of alcoholism, **American Journal of Orthopsychiatry, 51,** 489, 1981.
14. Cohn, V. H., New studies on the interaction of alcohol and cocaine, **Alcohol Health and Research World, 11**(4), 26, 1987.
15. Norton, R. and Noble, J., Combined alcohol and other drug use and abuse, **Alcohol Health and Research World, 11**(4), 78, 1987.
16. National Institute on Drug Abuse, **Annual Data 1985, Series 1**(5), DHHS #ADM86-1469, Alcohol, Drug Abuse, and Mental Health Administration, Rockville, Maryland, 1986.
17. Nace, E. P., **The Treatment of Alcoholism**, Brunner/Mazel, New York, 1987.
18. Radcliffe, A., Rush, P., Sites, C. F., and Cruse, J., **Pharmer's Almanac: Pharmacology of Drugs**, MAC Publishing, Denver, Colorado, 1989.
19. Lewis, J. A., Dana, R. Q., and Blevins, G. A., **Substance Abuse Counseling: An Individualized Approach**, Brooks/Cole, Pacific Grove, California, 1988.
20. Cohn, **New**, 1987.
21. Smith, D. E., Cocaine-alcohol abuse. Epidemiological, diagnostic and treatment consideration, **Journal of Psychoactive Drugs, 18,** 117, 1986.
22. Norton, **Combined**, 1987.
23. Baunach, P. J., Jail inmates, **Bureau of Justice Statistics Bulletin**, NCJ-99175, U. S. Department of Justice, Washington, D.

C., November 1983.

24. Trumble, J. G. and Walsh, J. M., A new initiative for solving age-old problems, **Alcohol Health and Research World, 9,** 2, 1985.

25. Braucht, G. N., Problem drinking among adolescents: A review and analysis of psychosocial research, in **Special Population Issues, Alcohol and Health, Monograph #4, National Institute on Alcohol Abuse and Alcoholism**, Rockville, Maryland, 1981.

26. Farber, E. D., The adolescent who runs, in **Youth At Risk for Substance Abuse,** Mills, A. R., Ed., DHHS # ADM87-1537. U. S. Government Printing Office, Washington, D. C. 1987.

27. Johnston, L. D., O'Malley, P. M. and Bachman, A. G., **1987 National High School Senior Drug Abuse Survey**, University of Michigan, Ann Arbor, Michigan, 1988.

28. Gerstein, D. R., Ed., **Toward the Prevention of Alcohol Problems: Government, Business and Community Action**, National Academy Press, Washington, D. C., 1984.

29. Hawkins, J. D., Lishner, D. M., Jenson, J. M., and Catalano, R. F. Jr., Delinquents and drugs: What the evidence suggests about prevention and treatment programming, in **Youth At High Risk For Substance Abuse**, Brown, B. W. and Mills, R., Eds., DHHS #ADM87-1537, U. S. Government Printing Office, Washington, D. C., 1987.

30. Arkin, **Communicating**, 1990.

31. Hartstone, E. and Hansen, K. V., The violent juvenile offender: An empirical portrait, in **Violent Juvenile Offenders: An Anthology**, Mathias, R. A., Demuro, P., and Allison, R. S., Eds., National Council on Crime and Delinquency, San Francisco, California, 1984.

32. Moore, D. and Siegel, H., Double trouble: Alcohol and other drug use among orthopedically impaired college students, **Alcohol Health and Research World, 13**(2), 119,

1989.

33. Moore, **Double**, 1989.

34. Cramer, S. L., Alcoholism and bullous changes of the lungs, **Alcohol Health and Research World, 13**, 166, 1989.

35. Zacny, J. P., Behavioral aspects of alcohol-tobacco interactions, **Recent Developments in Alcoholism, 8**, 205, 1990.

36. Kozlowski, L. T., Wilkinson, A., Skinner, W., Kent, C., Franklin, R., and Pope, M., Comparing tobacco cigarette dependence with other drug dependencies: Greater or equal 'difficulty quitting' and 'urges to use', but less 'pleasure' from cigarettes, **The Journal of the American Medical Association, 261**, 898, February 10, 1989.

37. Griffiths, R. R., Bigelow, G. E., and Liebson, I., Facilitation of human tobacco self-administration by ethanol: A behavioral analysis, **Journal of Experimental Analysis of Behavior, 25**, 279, 1976.

38. McCoy, G. D. and Napier, K., Alcohol and tobacco consumption as risk factors for cancer, **Alcohol Health and Research World, 10**, 28, 1986.

39. Phillips, D. K., Henderson, G. I., and Schenker, S., Pathogenesis of fetal alcohol syndrome, **Alcohol Health and Research World, 13**(3), 219, 1989.

40. Waterson, E. J. and Murray-Lyon, I. M. Drinking and smoking patterns amongst women attending an antenatal clinic, I. Before pregnancy, **Alcohol Health and Research World, 24**(2), 153, 1989.

41. Little, R. E., Moderate alcohol use during pregnancy and decreased infant birth weight, **American Journal of Public Health, 6**, 1154, 1977.

42. Phillips, **Pathogenesis**, 1989.

43. Sokol, R. J., Miller, S. I., and Reed, G. Alcohol abuse during pregnancy: An epidemiological study, Alcoholism: **Clinical and Experimental Research, 4**(2), 135, 1980.

44. Peacock, J. L., Bland, J. M., and Anderson, H. R., Effects on birthweight of alcohol and caffeine consumption in smoking women, **Journal of Epidemiology and Community Health, 45**(2), 159, 1991.

45. Nelson, D. J., Group helps smokers break addictive cycle, **Minneapolis Star Tribune, VIII**(53), 8, 1989.

46. Guenel, P., Chastang, J. F., and Luce, D., Leclerc, A., and Brugere, J., A study of the interaction of alcohol drinking and tobacco smoking among French cases of laryngeal cancer, **Journal of Epidemiology and Community Health, 42**(4), 350, 1988.

47. Rothman, K. J. and Keller, A., The effect of joint exposure to alcohol and tobacco on risk of cancer of the mouth and pharynx, **Journal of Chronic Diseases, 25**, 711, 1972.

48. Cann, C. I., Alcohol and cancer of the head and neck, **Alcohol Health and Research World, 10**(3), 34, 1986.

49. Rothman, **The effect**, 1972.

50. Orregia, F., DeStefani, E., Correa, P., and Fierro, L., Risk factors for cancer of the tongue in Uruguay, **Cancer, 67**(1), 180, 1991.

51. Zheng, T. Z., Boyle, P., Hu, H. F., Duan, J., Jiang, P. J., Ma, D. Q., Shui, L. P., Niu, S. R., and MacMahon, B., Tobacco smoking, alcohol consumption, and risk of oral cancer: A case-control study in Beijing, People's Republic of China, **Cancer, Causes, Control, 1**(2), 173, 1990.

52. Decker, J. and Goldstein, J. C., Risk factors in head and neck cancer, **New England Journal of Medicine, 306**, 1151, 1982.

Chapter 5

ALCOHOL AND NUTRITIONAL DEFICIENCIES

Alcohol affects an individual's nutritional state in a number of profound ways.[1] Specifically, alcohol contributes to nutritional deficiencies as seen in primary and secondary malnutrition.[2,3] **Primary malnutrition** occurs when alcohol displaces other foods from the diet and becomes the sole source of caloric (but not nutritional) needs. Heavy drinkers derive more than one-half of their daily energy or caloric needs from alcohol. **Secondary malnutrition** occurs when alcohol decreases the value of food by interfering with the digestion, absorption, transport, storage, and metabolism of various nutrients.

It appears that an inverse relationship exists between the intake of alcohol and the nutritional state of an individual. As the intake of alcohol increases, the percentage of energy derived from fat, protein and carbohydrates decreases. In addition, the intake of foods high in Vitamins A, C, and thiamin, or rich in calcium, fiber and iron also decline as a result of the increase in alcohol consumption.[4-7]

A number of studies have revealed that even moderate consumption of alcohol along with a healthy diet may still lead to liver damage.[8-11] Since the liver processes alcohol and breaks down toxic substances it is, therefore, the most susceptible organ to be damaged by alcohol ingestion. But in addition to alcohol damaging the liver, alcohol interferes with the liver's ability to metabolize nutrients and has a direct impact on nutrition and nutrient deprivation.[12-14] Therefore, to think that eating a healthy diet will offset any damage alcohol consumption can do to the body is a myth.

In addition to alcohol causing havoc with

the health of the adult drinker, adolescents also experience deleterious effects of alcohol. A report compiled through the Center for Disease Control revealed that 32 percent of teenage boys and 48 percent of teenage girls ate breakfast two or fewer days per week.[15] The typical teenage diet, which may substitute snack foods for foods rich in vitamins and minerals, together with the use of alcohol will negatively impact on the growth and development of the adolescent. At present little is known concerning the effects of alcohol on the nutritional well-being of adolescents. However, given the evidence derived from adult studies on alcohol and its impact on nutritional state of the individual, alcohol use among adolescents can only lead to adverse health consequences.[16]

I. VITAMINS

To maintain normal functioning of the body, certain complex chemicals or vitamins are essential. With the exception of Vitamin D, which is produced in the skin when exposed to sunlight, the body cannot manufacture vitamins and therefore, these substances must be obtained from the diet. Vitamins are categorized into fat or lipid-soluble and water-soluble vitamins.

A. Lipid or fat-soluble vitamins (A, D, E, and K) are absorbed with fats from the intestine into the blood and then stored in fatty tissue, principally the liver.

1. Vitamin A is essential for vision, reproduction and the maintenance of epithelia or cells that line body cavities. Vitamin A is required for protecting the linings of the respiratory, digestive, and urinary tracts against infection, and for healthy skin. Foods high in vitamin A are liver, carrots, dark leafy vegetables, yellow vegetables, fruits, particularly apricots, egg yolk, milk and dairy products, margarine, and carrots.[17,18]

Deficiency of Vitamin A may lead to night blindness, gonadal or sex gland dysfunction, weakening of the bones and teeth, and an increased risk of developing certain forms of cancer. Study has shown that many alcoholics have lower liver reserves of vitamin A.[19] Even in vitamin A rich diets, alcohol consumption contributed to a depletion of the liver's vitamin A stores.[20] Continued alcohol consumption and undetected vitamin A deficiency can result in any of the aforementioned physical consequences.

2. Vitamin D is essential for calcium and phosphate absorption from the intestine, and for the healthy growth of bones and teeth. Dietary sources of vitamin D are milk and other dairy products, fatty fish such as tuna, salmon, herring and sardines, liver, and egg yolk. Vitamin D is also produced in the skin when exposed to sunlight. Deficiency in vitamin D may result in bone disorders, such as rickets.

Alcohol consumption and vitamin D deficiency may be the result of either primary or secondary malnutrition. Alcohol intake may take precedence over eating foods rich in vitamin D or alcohol may interfere with the metabolism of vitamin D; primary and secondary malnutrition respectively. Several studies have identified vitamin D deficiency in alcoholics; e.g., decreased bone density,[21] decreased bone mass,[22] susceptibility to bone fractures,[23] and increased risk and incidence of osteoporosis.[24-26]

3. Vitamin E is essential for normal cell structure, helping prevent cell damage caused by chemical substances, maintaining the activities of certain enzymes, and for the formation of red blood cells. Vitamin E also protects red blood cells from being damaged or destroyed by toxins in the blood. Sources of food rich in Vitamin E are nuts, sunflower seeds, salad and cooking oils, green leafy vegetables, cereals, wheat germ, and egg yolk. Deficiency in vitamin E may lead to destruction of red blood cells, which may result in anemia.

Researchers have alleged that vitamin E deficiency in alcoholics may be due to primary malnutrition and liver disease.[27] Alcohol consumption together with a vitamin E deficient diet renders the liver even more susceptible to cell damage. Vitamin E deficiency is also associated with a neurologic syndrome characterized by neuromuscular weakness, motor incoordination in individuals with liver disease, and a lack of muscle coordination.[28]

4. **Vitamin K** is required for the proper coagulation of blood. Dietary sources rich in vitamin K are green leafy vegetables, especially cabbage, broccoli, lettuce, and turnip greens, vegetable oils, egg yolks, pork, liver, cheese, oats, wheat, rye and alfalfa.[29] Deficiency in vitamin K may result in delayed blood clotting, resulting in nosebleeds, bleeding gums, bleeding in the intestine and urinary tract. In severe cases, vitamin K deficiency may result in brain hemorrhage.[30] Although an inadequate intake of foods rich in vitamin K may not cause a clinical deficiency in alcoholics, blood clotting factors dependent on vitamin K drop "when alcohol-induced liver injury interferes with vitamin K utilization".[31]

B. **Water-soluble vitamins (C, B12, B6, Thiamin (B1), Riboflavin (B2), Folate or Folic Acid)** function as coenzymes, substances that assist enzymes in metabolic reactions. Deficiencies of water-soluble vitamins are more likely to occur than deficiencies of fat-soluble vitamins.

1. **Vitamin C** or ascorbic acid is necessary for maintenance of connective tissue, growth and maintenance of bones, teeth, gums, ligaments and blood vessels. Vitamin C is also essential for the metabolism of fats and certain amino acids, in healing wounds, and in the absorption of iron from the digestive tract. Dietary sources rich in vitamin C are citrus fruits, rose hips, green leafy vegetables, tomatoes, green peppers, strawberries, cantaloupe, onions, radishes, apples, pineapples, plums, peaches, and rutabagas.

Deficiency in vitamin C may result in scurvy, weak bones and loose teeth, anemia, nosebleeds and general weakness, aches and pains. At this time no definitive studies describe the negative relationship between alcohol consumption and vitamin C deficiency. However, if alcohol intake is displacing certain foods (primary malnutrition), it is likely that an individual with a moderate to high level of alcohol intake together with a diet deficient in vitamins may experience the consequences of vitamin C deficiency.

2. **Vitamin B12** functions as a coenzyme involved in carbohydrate and fat metabolism. It is essential in the production of red blood cells in bone marrow, utilization of folic acid, and in the functioning of the nervous system. Dietary sources of vitamin B12 are liver, kidney, beef, pork, chicken, fish, shellfish, eggs, and dairy products,

Deficiency in vitamin B12 may result in pernicious anemia, sore mouth and tongue. Vitamin B12 deficiency may also lead to depression, memory impairment and affect the nervous system and digestive track. Because the body has the ability to store greater amounts of vitamin B12, it may take several years before vitamin B12 deficiency symptoms appear. Therefore, alcoholics do not commonly suffer consequences as a result of vitamin B12 deficiency.[32]

3. Vitamin B6 (Pyridoxine) is a coenzyme primarily involved in amino acid metabolism. It is involved in the breakdown and utilization of carbohydrates, fats, and proteins, the manufacture of red blood cells, and in the functioning of the nervous and digestive systems. B6 is also important in the maintenance of healthy skin. Foods rich in vitamin B6 are rice, wheat bran, nuts, fish, meats, poultry, bananas, potatoes, and dried beans. Deficiency in vitamin B6 may cause weakness, irritability, skin disorders, inflammation of the mouth and tongue, anemia, and depression. "When alcoholism is not present, vitamin B6 deficiency is rare."[33] However, Lumeng and Li reported that low blood levels of vitamin B6 were present in more than 50 percent of alcoholics diagnosed with abnormal liver of blood function.[34]

4. Thiamin (B1) is a coenzyme necessary for cellular energy production. It is also involved in the breakdown and utilization of carbohydrates and in the functioning of the muscles, heart and nerves. Sources of Thiamin are whole grain cereals, legumes, leafy vegetables, meat, dairy products, brown rice, pasta, and nuts. Thiamin deficiency may result in cardiovascular, gastrointestinal, and nervous system disturbances. Mild thiamine deficiency may cause fatigue, loss of appetite, sleep disturbances, and irritability. Severe deficiency of Thiamine may result in beriberi (a disease characterized by polyneuritis, emaciation, and cardiac problems), constipation, abdominal pain, severe neurologic and cardiac complications, heart enlargement, rapid heartbeat, memory impairment, depression, and Wernicke-Korsakoff syndrome.[35,36]

Thiamin deficiency has been known to accompany alcoholism, and many alcoholics are at least mildly deficient in thiamin.[37,38] Thiamine deficiency in alcoholics may result in one of the many potentially disastrous physical and mental complications. Therefore, thiamin supplementation should be provided for individuals undergoing alcoholism treatment.[39]

5. Riboflavin (Vitamin B2) is a coenzyme involved in energy production and in the metabolism of amino acids, fatty acids, and carbohydrates. It is also essential in the utilization of other B vitamins, and in the production of hormones by the adrenal glands. Good sources of riboflavin are dairy products, eggs, organ meats such as liver, green leafy vegetables, whole grains, cereals and brewer's yeast. Riboflavin deficiency can result in mouth sores, chapped lips, dermatitis, eye disorders such as amblyopia (poor visual acuity) and photophobia (abnormal light sensitivity).[40]

Symptoms of riboflavin deficiency which include abnormalities in developing blood cells, and underdeveloped bone marrow have been identified in chronic alcoholics. Riboflavin deficiency also may result in anemia present in many alcoholics.[41]

6. Folate or Folic Acid assists enzymes that are involved in the synthesis of nucleic acids (the genetic material of cells). This vitamin also plays an important role in the production of red blood cells and in the healthy functioning of the nervous system. Foods containing folate are green leafy vegetables, egg yolk, organ meats such as liver, spinach, mushrooms, nuts, dried beans, peas, and whole-wheat bread. Folate deficiency affects those cells that divide the most rapidly and that are actively involved in nucleic acid synthesis. In addition, folate deficiency symptoms include anemia, mouth sores, and sore tongue.[42]

Researchers identified that as many as 38 percent of randomly selected alcoholics presented with low folate levels.[43] Feinman reported that "folate intake tends to be low in alcoholics who consume large amounts of alcohol".[44] Severe folate deficiency often resulted from a combination of low intake of foods rich in folic acid and impaired absorption which altered the structure and function of cells that line the intestine and shorten the intestinal villi. These changes subsequently impair the absorption of other nutrients such as sodium, glucose, water, and folate itself. As with thiamin deficiency, folate deficiency which is common in alcoholics, can be potentially disastrous. Vitamins replacing folate should be prescribed without hesitation.

II. MINERALS

Defined in nutrition, minerals are chemical elements that must be present in the diet for the proper and healthy functioning of the body. The following 13 minerals are essential for health - calcium, chromium, copper, fluorine, iodine, iron, magnesium, phosphorus, potassium, selenium, sodium, and zinc.

1. Calcium, the most abundant mineral in the body, is a major constituent of bones and teeth and represents approximately 85 percent of mineral matter in bones. Calcium is essential for the functioning of cells, muscle contraction, transmission of nerve impulses from nerve endings to muscle fibers, and blood clotting. Dietary sources high in calcium are dairy products, green leafy vegetables, fish, eggs, and fruit. Calcium deficiency can cause stunted growth or deformities of the bones and teeth. Symptoms of low calcium include muscle twitching, numbness, muscle spasms, seizures, and abnormal heart rhythms.

Hypocalcemia (low serum calcium) is common in individuals with severe alcoholism and liver disease. The association between alcoholism and low calcium levels may be due to either Vitamin D deficiency or diminished albumin (one of a group of simple proteins found in the blood) levels which in turn limit the amount of calcium that can remain dissolved in the blood.[45] Furthermore, abnormalities of bone metabolism found in alcoholics may be due to calcium malabsorption and requires further study.[46]

2. Iron is essential to life since it is essential to hemoglobin (red blood cell pigment) formation. "Iron is also present in enzymes that permit cellular respiration to occur".[47] Foods rich in iron include fish, eggs, meats, potatoes, grains, nuts, bean, green leafy vegetables, cauliflower, oysters, dandelions, and celery. Lack of iron can cause iron-deficiency anemia, lowered vitality, pale complexion, and decreased amount of hemoglobin in each red cell.

Both iron deficiency and iron excess have been documented in alcoholics. Regarding iron deficiency, researchers reported that alcoholics are often iron deficient as a result of gastrointestinal bleeding which is secondary to gastritis, duodenal ulcers, esophagitis, or cirrhosis, both caused by chronic alcohol consumption.[48,49]

Conversely, an excess of iron has also been reported in alcoholics. This increase in iron may result in damage to the liver and cause cirrhosis of the liver.[50] Excessive levels of iron is well documented in individuals with diagnosed alcoholic liver disease.[51] Approximately 29 percent of chronic alcohol drinkers actually have too much iron in their liver.[52]

3. Magnesium is essential for the formation of bones and teeth, transmission of nerve impulses, and for muscle contraction. It also assists enzymes that are involved in protein digestion and cellular energy production, and is associated with regulation of body temperature. Excellent sources of magnesium are soybeans, peanuts, nuts in general, whole grains, milk, seafood, and green leafy vegetables. Lack of magnesium in the diet may result in muscle spasms, central nervous system abnormalities, weakness, depression, and anxiety. There is also speculation that magnesium deficiency can lead to an increased risk of kidney stones or coronary heart disease.

Flink reported that low blood magnesium levels (hypomagnesemia) is a frequent and severe occurrence in alcoholics.[53] Low serum magnesium levels may be attributed to increased alcohol-induced urinary loss of magnesium, diarrhea, or vomiting.[54] Alcoholics may show symptoms of low blood levels of magnesium which include tremor, muscular twitches, muscle cramps, depression, confusion, apathy, abnormal heart rhythm, and cardiac arrest.[55] Chronic alcohol drinkers with low magnesium levels should be encouraged to replenish magnesium in their diets either through normal food intake sources or through magnesium supplements.

4. Zinc is a trace element that is required for the maintenance of healthy skin, bones, hair, normal growth, development of the reproductive organs, normal functioning of the prostate gland, healing of wounds, and the manufacture of nucleic acids (the genetic material of cells). Zinc also is an essential component of enzyme systems that are involved in digestion and respiration, and in the functioning of the hormone insulin. Dietary sources of zinc are beef, liver, peanuts, lamb, pork, wheat bran, poultry, cereals, seafood, and dried beans. Deficiency in zinc can result in loss of appetite, stunted growth, hair loss, skin, mouth, tongue and eyelid inflammation.

Alcoholics have been observed to have a frequent occurrence of low blood zinc levels and an increased urinary excretion of zinc.[56] Researchers have reported that individuals diagnosed with hepatitis or alcoholic cirrhosis of the liver had low blood zinc levels.[57-60] There is, however, speculation as to whether low blood zinc levels are attributable to chronic alcohol intake or as a result of liver disease.

Zinc deficiency is a frequent occurrence in alcoholics with or without liver disease. Whether zinc deficiency is a direct result of alcohol ingestion or due to liver disease, the fact remains that since chronic alcohol consumption significantly contributes to liver damage, zinc deficiency and complications therein, remains a significant factor for alcoholics. Manifestations of severe zinc deficiency in alcoholics include crusting skin lesions, hypogonadism (defective secretions of the sex glands) impaired night vision, depressed immune function, anorexia, impaired or depressed mental ability, birth defects as in Fetal Alcohol Syndrome (FAS).[61]

Researchers have also noted that zinc levels were significantly lower in alcoholic women than in non-alcohol drinking women.[62]

5. **Selenium** is a trace element that preserves the elasticity of body tissues, improves the oxygen supply to the heart and helps form prostaglandins. Prostaglandins are substances that help prevent high blood pressure and abnormal blood clotting. Selenium also interacts with vitamin E to protect cells against oxidation by toxic chemicals. Pro-longed selenium deficiency may cause pre-mature aging, muscle pain, heart disease, and abnormalities of skeletal and heart muscles.[63] Dietary sources high in selenium are brazil nuts, seafood, butter, meat, and whole grains.

Recent studies have identified that low blood selenium levels have been observed in alcoholics with or without liver disease.[64-66] Therefore, low blood selenium levels leave the chronic alcohol drinker vulnerable to any of the complications caused by selenium deficiency.

III. AMINO ACIDS

In addition to depleting the body of necessary vitamins and minerals or distorting their normal levels of absorption, as in the body absorbing excessive amounts of iron, chronic alcohol consumption also causes amino acid abnormalities. Amino acids are the building blocks on which proteins are constructed and are the end-products of protein digestion. Clinicians have found that it is common for alcoholics to have amino acid abnormalities. Amino acid abnormalities have also been linked with portal-systemic encephalopathy (PSE). PSE, also known as hepatic encephalopathy, is a dysfunction of the brain associated with liver disease and characterized by impaired intellectual functioning, behavioral and personality changes, and neuromuscular disturbances. Persons afflicted with PSE may experience changes in consciousness from mild disorientation to coma. Since amino acid abnormalities have been identified in alcoholics, PSE is a serious and debilitating consequence of chronic alcohol consumption. [67]

1. Tryptophan an essential amino acid necessary for normal growth and development and a precursor of serotonin, whose functions are associated with mood, has also been found in decreased levels in alcoholics.[68] Researchers have indicated that low levels of serotonin in the brain may be the cause of increased or frequent states of aggression or depression often observed in alcoholics.[69]

IV. GLUCOSE

The body's chief source of energy and the most important carbohydrate in body metabolism is glucose. It is formed during digestion and absorbed from the intestines into the blood of the portal vein. Excess glucose is converted into glycogen when it passes through the liver. Glycogen's principal role is in controlling blood sugar levels. When blood sugar levels are low, glycogen is converted back to glucose.

Two conditions that may be induced by alcohol consumption that disturb normal levels of glucose are hypoglycemia (low blood sugar) and hyperglycemia (increased blood sugar).[70] Hypoglycemia as a result of alcohol-induced fasting is a dangerous disorder and is found in chronically malnourished individuals. Alcohol-induced hypoglycemia must be diagnosed and treated early or the consequence can be fatal. Symptoms of alcohol-induced hypoglycemia include fatigue, weakness, delirium, coma, and if left untreated, death. Administration of intravenous glucose is required for the individual experiencing low blood sugar symptoms. Once the individual responds to glucose injections, only modest levels of carbohydrates are necessary to prevent a relapse.[71,72]

Researchers have reported that alcohol-induced hypoglycemia may also occur in well nourished alcohol drinkers who eat a low carbohydrate diet and engage in strenuous physical activity or exercise.[73,74]

In a review of research studies pertaining to alcohol-induced hyperglycemia, Patel reported conflicting results.[75] Whereas some researchers observed moderate levels of alcohol ingestion contributing to hyperglycemia, other researchers reported no noticeable effect on glucose levels after ingestion of alcohol in low to moderate doses (equal to two glasses of sherry).[76,77] However, consumption of larger doses of alcohol (266 to 513 ml, consumed over 1 to 3 days) resulted in glucose intolerance in both normal individuals and subjects diagnosed with diabetes. Although alcohol-induced hyperglycemia is not as serious as alcohol-induced hypoglycemia, in severe cases hyperglycemia can cause confusion and coma.[78]

In pregnancy, glucose levels are very important in the growth and development of the unborn child. Glucose is the primary fuel for the developing fetus, and consequently, low glucose may be a factor linked to Fetal Alcohol Syndrome (FAS).[79,80]. (FAS is discussed in greater detail in Chapter 1). Researchers have also found a positive correlation between glucose disturbances and brain growth abnormalities in the developing fetus.[81] Hypoglycemia has been positively linked with fetal growth retardation in mothers who consumed alcohol during pregnancy.[82,83]

V. LIPIDS, FATS, AND FATTY ACIDS

Lipids are a group of fatty substances that include triglycerides (the principal form of fat in body fat and a source of energy), phospholipids (a type of fat found in all cells that form the structural basis of cell membranes), and cholesterol (an important component of the cell membrane).[84] Reitz noted that biochemical changes and alterations in the lipid profile of various organs and blood cells were apparent in alcoholics and in animals exposed to ethanol.[85]

Hyperlipidemia is a condition caused by chronic alcohol consumption in which the blood contains higher than normal levels of fats or lipids. When too many fats are produced, the result may be liver disease. Fats may either be stored in the liver thereby damaging it or released into the blood as triglycerides and cholesterol which in turn can lead to heart disease or stroke. Studies have documented that increased levels of fats in the blood increases the risk of hardening of the arteries and heart disease.[86]

Some studies have shown that alcohol ingested in small quantities (one to two drinks per day) can increase the blood level of HDL (high density lipoprotein) which may protect against heart disease.[87] Rifkind cited evidence that supported the theory that the HDL levels in blood cholesterol protected against coronary artery disease by removing fatty deposits from the blood vessels. Consequently, since alcohol consumption raises HDL levels, it is plausible that alcohol can protect against the incidence of coronary artery disease.[88]

However, Hurt and associates have reported that there is more than one type of HDL cholesterol and alcohol has no effect on HDL2, the type which is regarded to be protective against coronary artery disease.[89] In addition, several studies have refuted the hypothesis that alcohol does protect against coronary artery disease. Although the overall evidence is suggestive, researchers contend that recommending alcohol for therapeutic use is premature since concrete documentation has not yet established that alcohol protects against coronary artery disease or cardiovascular disease.[90,91] Evidence of hyperlipidemia in chronic alcohol drinkers appears to contradict postulated evidence that alcohol drinking is associated with HDL thereby lowering the risk of heart disease. Taking other steps to prevent heart disease, such as exercising, not smoking, and eating a low-fat diet, far outweigh alcohol's potential benefits of preventing heart disease. The numerous documented health problems and accidents caused by alcohol consumption

126 ALCOHOL AND NUTRITIONAL DEFICIENCIES

present a much stronger case for abstinence than drinking a glass or two of wine for "medicinal purposes".

SUMMARY

Alcohol use and abuse affects an individual's nutritional state either through primary or secondary malnutrition. Primary malnutrition occurs when alcohol becomes the sole source of caloric needs and replaces other foods in a person's diet. Secondary malnutrition occurs when the value of food is decreased due to alcohol's interference in the proper digestion, transport, storage, or metabolism of nutrients. An inverse relationship exists between alcohol intake and the nutritional state of the individual. The higher the alcohol intake, the lower the percentage of energy derived from fat, protein or carbohydrates.

The following is a summary of the adverse health consequences on the nutritional state caused by chronic alcohol use:

DEFICIENCY IN   ADVERSE CONSEQUENCES

Fat-soluble vitamins
    Vitamin A   Night blindness
                            Gonadal dysfunction
                            Weak bones, teeth
                            Increased risk of cancers
    Vitamin D   Decreased bone density
                            Decreased bone mass
                            Bone fractures
                            Risk of osteoporosis
    Vitamin E   Liver cell damage
                            Neuromuscular weakness
                            Motor incoordination
                            Lack of muscle coordination
    Vitamin K   Impaired blood clotting

Water Soluble Vitamins

Vitamin C	May result in scurvy, weak bones, loose teeth, nosebleeds
	General weakness, aches, pains
Vitamin B12	Alcoholics do not commonly suffer consequences of B12 deficiency
Vitamin B6	Anemia
	Irritability
	Depression
	Skin Disorders
Thiamin (B1)	Cardiovascular disturbances
	Gastrointestinal disturbances
	Nervous system disturbances
Riboflavin (B2)	Anemia
	Underdeveloped bone marrow
Folate or Folic Acid	Altered structure and function of cells that line the intestine and shorten intestinal villi.

Minerals

Calcium	Hypocalcemia
Iron	Excess of iron in alcoholics causes damage to liver and cirrhosis
Magnesium	Hypomagnesemia
	Tremor
	Muscular twitches, cramps
	Depression
	Confusion, apathy
	Abnormal heart rhythm
	Cardiac arrest
Zinc	Crusting skin lesions
	Hypogonadism
	Impaired night vision
	Depressed immune function

	Anorexia
	Impaired mental ability
	Birth defects (e.g., FAS)
Selenium	Premature aging
	Muscle pain
	Heart disease
	Abnormalities of skeletal and heart muscles
Amino Acids	Port systemic encephalopathy (PSE)
Tryptophan	Depression
	Increased aggression
Glucose	Hypoglycemia
	Hyperglycemia
	Brain growth abnormalities in developing fetus
	Fetal growth retardation
Lipids, Fats, Fatty Acids	Hyperlipidemia

Unfortunately, eating a healthy diet will not offset any damage caused by alcohol abuse. Chronic alcohol use will have a deleterious effect on the proper digestion, transport, storage, and metabolism of vitamins, minerals, amino acids, glucose, and lipids, fats, and fatty acids. Despite the fact that alcohol in many cases displaces healthy foods, it ranks slightly lower than eggshells and coffee grounds in nutritional value.[92]

REFERENCES

1. Mendoza, T., Very distant relatives: Alcohol and nutrition, **Current Health, 20**, October 2, 1990.

2. Feinman, L., Absorption and utilization of nutrients in alcoholism, **Alcohol Health**

and Research World, 13(3), 207, 1989.

3. Lieber, C. S., Alcohol and nutrition. **Alcohol Health and Research World, 13**(3), 197, 1989.

4. Gruchow, H. W., Sobocinski, K. A., Barboriak, J. J., and Scheller, J. G., Alcohol consumption, nutrient intake and relative body weight among U. S. adults, **American Journal of Clinical Nutrition, 42**(2), 189, 1985.

5. Hillers, V. N. and Massey, L. K., Interrelationships of moderate and high alcohol consumption with diet and health status, **American Journal of Clinical Nutrition, 41**(2), 356, 1986.

6. Lieber, **Alcohol**, 1989.

7. Sherlock, S., Nutrition and the alcoholic, **Lancet, 1**(8374), 436, 1984.

8. Lieber, C. S., Alcohol and the liver: Overview, in **Recent Developments in Alcoholism**, Galante, M., Ed., Plenum Press, New York, 1984.

9. Lieber, C. S., Jones, D. P., Mendelson, J., and DeCarli, L. M., Fatty liver, hyperlipidemia and hyperuricemia produced by prolonged alcohol consumption despite adequate dietary intake, **Transactions of the Association of American Physicians, 76**, 289, 1963.

10. Lieber, C. S., Jones, D. P., and DeCarli, L. M., Effects of prolonged ethanol intake: Production of fatty liver despite adequate diets, **Journal of Clinical Investigations, 44**, 1009, 1965.

11. Lieber, C. S. and Rubin, E., Alcoholic fatty liver in man on a high protein and low fat diet, **American Journal of Medicine, 44**(2), 200, 1968.

12. Lieber, **Alcohol**, 1989.

13. Mendoza, **Very distant relatives**, 1990.

14. Rothschild, M. A., Oratz, M., and Schreiber, S. S., Alcohol-induced liver disease: Does nutrition play a role? **Alcohol Health and Research World, 13**, 228, 1989.

15. Center for Disease Control, Association for the Advancement of Health Education (CDC),

Results from the national adolescent student health survey, **Journal of the American Medical Association, 261**(14), 2025, 1989.

16. Arria, A. M., Tarter, R. E., and Van Thiel, D. J., The effects of alcohol abuse on the health of adolescents, **Alcohol Health and Research World, 15**(1), 52, 1991.

17. Clayman, C. B., Ed., **The American Medical Association: Encyclopedia of Medicine**, Random House, New York, 1989.

18. National Cancer Institute (NCI), Vitamins and minerals, **Alcohol Health and Research World, 13**(3), 238, 1989.

19. Leo, M. A. and Lieber, C. S., Alcohol and Vitamin A, **Alcohol Health and Research World, 13**(3), 250, 1989.

20. Leo, **Alcohol**, 1989.

21. Saville, P. D., Changes in bone mass with age and alcoholism, **Journal of Bone and Joint Surgery, 47**, 492, 1965.

22. Gascon-Barre, M. and Joly, J. G., The biliary excretion of (3H)-25-hydroxy-vitamin D3 following chronic ethanol administration in the rat, **Life Sciences, 28**, 279, 1981.

23. Nilsson, B. E., Conditions contributing to fracture of the femoral neck, **Acta Chirurgica Scandinavica, 136**(5), 383, 1970.

24. Larkin, M., Nutrient snatchers: It isn't only our vices that can rob our bodies of vitamins and minerals, **Mature Health, 24**, November 1989.

25. Solomon, L., Drug induced arthropathy and necrosis of the femoral head, **Journal of Bone and Joint Surgery, 55**(2), 246, 1973.

26. Lieber, **Alcohol**, 1989.

27. Tanner, A. R., Bantock, I., Hinks, L., Lloyd, B., Turner, N.R., and Wright, R., Depressed selenium and vitamin E levels in an alcoholic population: Possible relationship to hepatic injury through increased lipid peroxidation, **Digestive Diseases and Sciences, 31**(12), 1307, 1986.

28. Sokol, R. J., Iannaccone, S. T., Bove, K. E., and Heubi, J. E., Vitamin E deficiency

neurologic syndrome during chronic cholestasis: Beneficial effects of early alpha-tocopherol therapy, **Oediatric Research, 17,** 367, 1983.

29. Thomas, C. L., Ed., **Taber's Cyclopedic Medical Dictionary**, 16th Ed., F. A. Davis, Philadelphia, PA, 1989.

30. Clayman, **American Medical**, 1989.

31. Lieber, **Alcohol**, 1989, p. 201.

32. Lieber, **Alcohol**, 1989.

33. NCI, **Vitamins**, 1989.

34. Lumeng, L. and Li, T. K., Vitamin B6 metabolism in chronic alcohol abuse: Pyridoxal phosphate levels in plasma and the effects of acetaldehyde on pyridoxal phosphate synthesis and degradation in human erythrocytes, **Journal of Clinical Investigation, 53**(3), 693, 1974.

35. Lieber, **Alcohol**, 1989.

36. Mendoza, **Very distant**, 1990.

37. Feinman, **Absorption**, 1989.

38. Leevy, C. M., Baker, H., Ten Hove, W., Frank, O., and Cherrick, G. R., B-complex vitamin in liver disease of the alcoholic, **American Journal of Clinical Nutrition, 16,** 339, 1965.

39. Lieber, **Alcohol**, 1989.

40. Thomas, **Taber's**, 1989.

41. National Institute on Alcohol Abuse and Alcoholism (NIAAA), Medical consequences of alcohol, Special focus: The fifth special report to the U. S. Congress on alcohol and health. **Alcohol Health and Research World, 9**(1), 19, 1984.

42. Thomas, **Taber's**, 1989.

43. World, M. J., Ryle, P. R., John, D. J., Shaw, G. K., and Thompson, A. D., Differential effect of chronic alcohol intake and poor nutrition on body weight and fat stores, **Alcohol ad Alcoholism, 19**(4), 281, 1984.

44. Feinman, **Absorption**, 1989.

45. Marsano, L. and McClain, C. J., Effects of alcohol on electrolytes and minerals, **Alcohol Health and Research World, 13**(3), 255, 1989.

46. Feinman, **Absorption**, 1989.
47. Thomas, **Taber's**, 1989.
48. Feinman, **Absorption**, 1989.
49. Marsano, **Effects**, 1989.
50. Clayman, **American Medical**, 1989.
51. Marsano, **Effects**, 1989.
52. Lieber, **Alcohol**, 1989.
53. Flink, E. B., Magnesium deficiency in alcoholism, **Alcoholism: Clinical and Experimental Research, 10**(6), 590, 1986.
54. Feinman, **Absorption**, 1989.
55. Marsano, **Effects**, 1989.
56. Lieber, **Alcohol**, 1989.
57. Hartoma, T. R., Sotaniemi, E. A., Pelkonen, O., and Ahlqvist, J., Serum zinc and serum copper and indices of drug metabolism in alcoholics, **European Journal of Clinical Pharmacology, 12**, 147, 1977.
58. Smith, J. C. Jr., Brown, E. D., White, S. C., and Finkelstein, J. D., Plasma vitamin A and zinc concentration in patients with alcoholic cirrhosis, **Lancet, 1**(7918), 1975.
59. Sullivan, J. F., Williams, R. V., and Burch, R. E., The metabolism of zinc and selenium in cirrhotic patients during six weeks of zinc ingestion, **Alcoholism: Clinical and Experimental Research, 3**, 235, 1979.
60. Valberg, L. S., Flanagan, P. R., Ghent, C. N., and Chamberlain, M. J., Zinc absorption and leucocyte zinc in alcoholic and non-alcoholic cirrhosis, **Digestive Diseases and Sciences, 30**(4), 329, 1985.
61. Marsano, **Effects**, 1989.
62. Flynn, A., Martier, S. S., Sokol, R. J., Miller, S. I., Golden, N. L., and Villano, B. C., Zinc status of pregnant alcoholic women: A determinant of fetal outcome, **Lancet, 1**(8220), 572, 1981.
63. Marsano, **Effects**, 1989.
64. Dutta, S. K., Miller, P. A., Greenberg, L. B., and Levander, O. A., Selenium and acute alcoholism, **American Journal of Clinical Nutrition, 38**(5), 713, 1983.
65. Dworkin, B., Rosenthal, W. S.,

Jankowski, R. H., Gordon, G. G., and Haldea, D., Low blood selenium levels in alcoholics with and without advanced liver disease: Correlations with clinical and nutritional status, **Digestive Diseases and Sciences, 30**(9), 838, 1985.

66. Valimaki, M. J., Harju, K. J., and Ylikarhri, R. H., Decreased serum selenium in alcoholics: A consequence of liver dysfunction, **Clinical Chimica Acta, 130**(3), 291, 1983.

67. Lieber, **Alcohol**, 1989, 202.

68. Lieber, **Alcohol**, 1989.

69. Branchey, L., Branchey, M., Shaw, S., and Lieber, C. S., Relationship between changes in plasma amino acids and depression in alcoholic patients, **American Journal of Psychiatry, 141**(10), 1212, 1984.

70. Gloeckner, **From drinking**, 1990.

71. Madison, L. L., Ethanol induced hypoglycemia, in **Advances in Metabolic Disorders**, Vol. 3, Levine, R. and Luft, R., Eds., Academic Press, New York. 1968.

72. Patel, D. G., Effects of ethanol on carbohydrate metabolism and implications for the aging alcoholic, **Alcohol Health and Research World, 13**(3), 240, 1989.

73. Haight, J. S. J. and Keatings, W. R., Failure of thermoregulation in the cold during hypoglycemia induced by exercise and ethanol, **Journal of Physiology, 229**, 87, 1973.

74. McLaughlan, J. M., Joel, F. J., and Moodie, C. A., Hypoglycemia in humans induced by alcohol and a low carbohydrate diet, **Nutrition Reports International, 8**(5) 331, 1973.

75. Patel, **Effects**, 1989.

76. Phillips, G. B. and Safrit, S. P., Alcoholic diabetes: Induction of glucose intolerance with alcohol, **Journal of the American Medical Association, 217**(11), 1513, 1979.

77. Shanley, B. C., Robertson, E. J., Joubert, S. M., ad Morth-Goombes, J. D.,

134   ALCOHOL AND NUTRITIONAL DEFICIENCIES

Effects of alcohol on glucose intolerance, **Lancet, 1**, 1232, 1972.

78. Patel, **Effects**, 1989.

79. Freinkel, N., Banting Lecture 1980, Of pregnancy and progeny, **Diabetes, 29**(12), 1023, 1980.

80. Freinkel, N., Lewis, N. J., Akazawa, S., Roth, S. I., and Gorman, L., The honeybee syndrome - implications of the teratogenicity of mannose in rat-embryo culture, **New England Journal of Medicine, 310**(4), 223, 1984.

81. Singh, S. P., Pullen, G. L., and Snyder, A. K., Effects of ethanol on fetal fuels and brain growth in rats, **Journal of Laboratory and Clinical Medicine, 112**(6), 704, 1988.

82. Gruppuso, P. A., Migliori, R., Susa, J. B., and Schwarts, R., Chronic maternal hyperinsulinemia and hypoglycemia. A model for experimental intrauterine growth retardation, **Biology Neonate, 40**(3-4), 113, 1981.

83. Nitzen, M., Relation between maternal and fetal blood glucose levels in experimental intrauterine growth retardation, **Israel Journal of Medical Science, 17**(5), 373, 1981.

84. Salem, N. Jr., Alcohol, fatty acids, and diet, **Alcohol Health and Research World, 13**(3), 211, 1989.

85. Reitz, R. C., The effects of ethanol ingestion on lipid metabolism, **Progress in Lipid Research, 18**(12), 87, 1979.

86. Gloeckner, **From drinking**, 1990.

87. Mendoza, **Very distant**, 1990.

88. Rifkind, B. W., High-density lipoprotein cholesterol and coronary artery disease: Survey of the evidence, **American Journal of Cardiology, 66**, 3A, 1990.

89. Hurt, R. D., Briones, E. R., Offord, K. P., Patton, J. G., Mao, S. J., Morse, R. M., and Kottke, B. A., Plasma lipids and apolipoprotein A-I and A-II levels in chronic patients, **American Journal of Clinical Nutrition, 43**(4), 521, 1986.

90. Klatsky, A. L., Alcohol and coronary

artery disease, **Alcohol Health and Research World, 14**(4), 289, 1990.

91. Lands, W. E. M. and Zakhari, S., Alcohol and cardiovascular disease, **Alcohol Health and Research World, 14**(4), 304, 1990.

92. Gloeckner, **From drinking**, 1990.

Chapter 6

ALCOHOLISM AND THE FAMILY

Researchers contend that children of alcoholics are one of the highest at-risk populations for developing alcoholism as well as behavioral and emotional problems.[1-9] An estimated 28 million individuals over the age of 18 are children of alcoholics, and some 7 million children under the age of 18 are living in alcoholic families.[10] Tables 6.1 and 6.2 illustrate the problems experienced by the alcoholic's family as reported in research. These findings encapsulate the current under-standing of the effect of parental alcoholism on the child.

Table 6.1

Alcohol-Related Problems Experienced By Drinker and His/Her Family Members

- Family and Marital Conflict
- Child and Spouse Abuse
- Increased Divorce Rate
- Loss of Self-Esteem for Drinker and Family
- Physical and/or Mental Complications
- Job Performance Affected
- Legal Problems
- Fetal Damage from Maternal Drinking
- Child Rearing Problems Resulting in
    Neglect
    Child Development Problems
    Juvenile Drinking
    Juvenile Delinquency

Table 6.2

**Problems Experienced by Children
Who Live in Alcoholic Homes**

<u>Neglect or Abuse of the Child</u>
    -Physical and/or emotional neglect
    -Physical, emotional, and/or sexual abuse
    -Accidents
    -Physical health affected
    -Psychosomatic illnesses

<u>Conduct Problems</u>
    -Delinquency
    -Police and court involvement
    -Aggression or acting out behaviors
    -School work affected
    -School failure
    -Alcohol and drug abuse
    -Sexual activity

<u>Vulnerability to Emotional Problems</u>
    -Depression
    -Suicidal ideation and/or attempts
    -Lack of self-confidence, self-worth, or self-esteem
    -Fear of abandonment
    -Post-Traumatic Stress Disorder as a result of experiencing or witnessing physical, emotional or sexual abuse
    -Anxiety
    -Repressed anger or hostility
    -Hypersensitivity

<u>Difficulties With Interpersonal Relationships</u>
    -Family relationship problems due to unclear parental and child roles or confused family boundaries
    -Problems with peer relationships
    -Adjustment problems
    -Feeling different from everyone else
    -Feeling overresponsible
    -Inability to trust others

I. Alcoholic Children of Alcoholics

Drew, Moon and Buchanan contended that one of the highest at-risk populations for developing alcoholism is children of alcoholics. In their study, they found that 30 percent of alcoholics had a parent who was alcoholic, 5 percent of alcoholics had parents who were moderate drinkers, and 10 percent of alcoholics had parents who were abstainers.[11] Researchers have identified and confirmed that adult children of alcoholics are at a significantly higher risk of becoming alcoholics than children of non-alcoholic parents.[12-18] Beardslee, Son and Vaillant found that children who lived in alcoholic homes where they experienced a disorganized and discordant life, were at a greater risk for developing alcoholism as adults.[19]

In studies where male and female alcoholics were compared, researchers consistently reported that female alcoholics were more likely to have an alcoholic parent and/or family members.[20-22] Estimates of incidence of paternal alcoholism were higher for alcoholic women then men, but both male and female alcoholics were equally likely to have an alcoholic mother.[23]

Although there is a lack of consensus as to what specifically may predispose an individual in becoming an alcoholic, genetics research has strengthened the evidence that links alcoholism to the transmission of particular traits or genes. Although genes do not directly cause alcoholism, genes can influence certain behaviors indirectly by increasing an individual's vulnerability for alcoholism. Research studies have revealed that alcoholism may be linked to the central and peripheral nervous systems. However, it is not yet clear how these factors contribute to the development of alcoholism.[24]

The strongest evidence for the transmission

of alcoholism as a "family disease" has been in the area of twins and adopted-out sibling studies.[25] Researchers have demonstrated that the frequency of alcoholism among identical twins was higher than among fraternal twins.[26,27] Identical or monozygotic twins have 100 percent genetic likeness, and fraternal or dizygotic twins have only 50 percent genetic likeness. Fraternal twins are no more similar than siblings born at different times to the same parents. In a study conducted with 174 male pairs of twins, alcohol abuse was identified in 54 percent of the identical twins, as compared to 28 percent rate of alcohol abuse among fraternal twins.[28] Overall, twin studies have supported the premise that substantial genetic influence exists in predisposing an individual to alcoholism.

Adoption studies have also supported the belief of genetic predisposition to alcoholism. Evidence collected through adoption studies has suggested that a genetic predisposition to alcoholism was a stronger determinant to the development of alcoholism than parental rearing practices in the adoptive home.[29-32]

Pertaining to women and alcoholism, it was found that when compared with men, women were more likely to abuse alcohol when faced with a particular problem or distressing life situation. Researchers in the field of women and alcoholism have consistently reported that problem drinking appears to correlate positively with specific life situations and psychological stress experienced by the woman.[33-35] Another finding in studies concerning alcohol abuse among women relates to communication between family members. Wilson has stated that an atmosphere of silence and tension appears to be a common finding among families of alcohol abusing daughters. There was not only a lack of communication between the drinking members of the family but a lack of communication between any of the members of the family.[36]

II. EMOTIONAL EFFECTS OF PARENTAL ALCOHOLISM ON OFFSPRING:

The high risk of alcoholism is but one of the deleterious effects of being raised in an alcoholic home. Children of alcoholics are also at risk for developing emotional and behavioral problems due to the continuous stress and conflict experienced by these youngsters. In a study conducted of 115 children of alcoholics between the ages of 10 and 15, Cork reported that 56 of these children experienced emotional damage that was considered fairly serious and 50 children experienced very serious emotional damage.
In the same study, 113 children felt their relationships within the family affected, and 111 children felt that their relationships outside of the family were affected.[37]

Researchers claim that the unpredictable and chaotic behavior of alcoholic families hinders the proper emotional development of the child.[38-40] The developing personality of the child is "adversely affected when parents show extremely deviant behavior associated with alcoholism."[41] Research findings suggest that children of alcoholics present problems in personality development and identity formation, serious psychosocial illnesses which are associated with parental alcoholism, and an increased psychopathology.[42-44]

West and Prinz reported that children of alcoholics presented greater degrees of various mental disorders than did children reared in nonalcoholic homes.[45] Children reared in alcoholic homes presented both internalizing and externalizing disorders. Internalizing disorders refer to various levels of depression and anxiety. Externalizing disorders refer to acting out behaviors such as conduct problems and aggression. Furthermore, the degree of dysfunction or level of emotional distress in children of alcoholics appeared to be related to the severity of the father's drinking problem.[46,47]

In regard to adult children of alcoholics, researchers concluded that more antisocial behaviors and episodes of uncontrollable anger were found among adult children of alcoholics than among adults from nonalcoholic families.[48,49] Conduct problems in particular were found to be highly associated with parental alcoholism.[50] Another strong relationship was found between anxiety in adult children of alcoholics and parental alcoholism.[51-53] Researchers have also demonstrated a greater susceptibility to depression among young and adult children of alcoholics, especially among females.[54-56]

III. FAMILY VIOLENCE

Researchers in the area of violence in the family suggest that both victims of abuse and witnesses to violent behaviors within the family are at greater risk for developing psychological problems.[57-61] It was concluded that children exposed to anger reacted with various signs of distress which ranged from crying to acts of aggression.

The most significant aspect of being a victim or witnessing an act of aggression toward a family member is the following: The threat of physical harm, whether personal or toward a family member, provokes the most intense of human reactions and leaves an emotional imprint, which often lasts a lifetime.[62] This emotional imprint may manifest itself as post-traumatic stress disorder and is more severe when the stressor is of human design.[63]

Putnam, Post and Guroff stated that the difference between the child who was a direct victim of abuse as compared with the child who witnessed abusive behaviors is in the subsequent psychopathology manifested by the child. Whereas the "victim" may have dissociative symptoms which encompass psychogenic amnesia[2], the "witness" may have full recall of the distressing event.[64] Despite this difference between "victims" and "witnesses", children of alcoholics who experience severe emotional, physical or sexual abuse (directly or indirectly) may manifest symptoms of post-traumatic stress disorder due to the intensity and duration of the abusive behaviors exhibited by the parent(s) in the alcoholic family.

IV. STRESS ASSOCIATED WITH PARENTAL ALCOHOLISM

The area of family stress is an area that has received wide attention in relation to children raised in alcoholic families. All families, regardless of alcoholism experience stress. However, a healthy family adjusts to stress and the crisis is seen as temporary with the family members maintaining their appropriate roles of parents or children. Bell identified that "well families adopt mechanisms which actually resolve discrepancies or at least contain them in ways that are not pathogenic for individual members."[65] In contrast, in an alcoholic family the fluctuations between critical and noncritical situations oscillate dramatically, inconsistently and chaotically. The child of the alcoholic must therefore, "on a day-to-day basis, accommodate change that is both sudden and sharp, not merely on the part

---

[2] **Psychogenic amnesia** denotes the sudden inability to recall important personal information and is not due to organic or physical causes (**DSM-III-R**).

of the alcoholic parent but usually both parents."[66]

Whether healthy or dysfunctional, the family is the main source of the individual's belief and value systems and codes of behavior that ultimately determine the individual's understanding of the world and his/her place in it.[67] In fact, the defining functional characteristic of the family is the socialization of children.[68] The mental health of the individual, therefore, is related to the explicit or implicit teachings of the family and the offspring's interpretation of these "teachings" along with the interpretation of meanings of family role models, and relationships among family members and the family members' connection to and interaction with the world in general.

Since the family is the first group that has a major impact on the development of the child, and it has been contended by researchers that the alcoholic family has a debilitating impact on the child due to the continuous stress within the family, it is important to get a clear understanding as to what impact stress may have on _any_ family system, regardless of whether it may be termed as healthy or dysfunctional. Once we have this understanding, we can then look at what makes an alcoholic family different based on research findings on the following dimensions:

    a. how the alcoholic family deals with stress.
    b. what constitutes stress within the alcoholic family, and
    c. how offspring learn to deal with stress within the immediate family and in adult years as well.

Stress within the family is an important variable to understand since it hinges directly on the research findings of alcoholism and drug abuse as well as emotional and behavioral problems manifested by children of alcoholics. For example, alcoholism among children of alcoholics may be one of the coping strategies "learned" in alcoholic families when dealing with stress.

Lazarus defined stress as a "whole area of problems that includes stimuli producing stress reactions, the reactions themselves, and the various intervening processes."[69] Thus, stress encompasses physiological, psychological and sociological phenomena. McCubbin, Cauble and Patterson divide stressors into two categories: normative (naturally occurring) and nonnormative (unexpected).[70]

Normative stressors include all naturally occurring developmental phenomena that are predictable over the life span of individuals and families as well. Normative stressors may include Erik Erikson's psychosocial stages of human development: prenatal to infancy, infancy to childhood, childhood to adolescence, adolescence to adulthood, adulthood to old age, and old age to death.[71] Normative stressors also include events peculiar to the family unit itself, such as marriage, birth of first child, families with adolescents, retirement, etc.

Nonnormative stressors include all unanticipated family events that place the family members in a stage of flux and instability. Unanticipated events may be a sudden illness in the family, loss of employment, etc. Since families are not usually prepared for nonnormative stressors, they are not prepared to cope "and may not have available the social, psychological, or material resources needed to manage such events."[72]

At present there are two positions as to how a family may emerge when faced with nonnormative stressors. The first position contends that a crisis may provide an
as family members move toward greater maturity and increased mental health. The second oppor-

tunity for growth through morphogenesis[3] position suggests that a potentially dysfunctional family unit may adopt negative or unhealthy coping strategies, such as alcohol or drug use, which tend to be reinforced within the family and become part of the family's coping strategy repertoire.[73]

On the whole, researchers have concluded that the alcoholic family is a system of ongoing trauma in which a series of ongoing crises bring the family to a catastrophic state.[74,75] Eventually the family members learn to cope with chronic stress which has become the norm within the alcoholic family.[76]

Coping refers to any behaviors or cognitive strategies that individuals may adopt in order to reduce harm or threat presented by a situation. Initially, coping strategies in response to a crisis are not a natural part of an individual's or family's basic repertoire and involve the integration of psychological and sociological frameworks.[77] In terms of psychological coping strategies, Lazarus emphasized both direct actions and palliative or alleviating psychic pain strategies.[78]

Direct or **active coping strategies** refer to those behaviors that are overt in nature such as "fight or flight" responses. These responses or behaviors attempt to alter or outwardly change the harmful, threatening or painful situation. For example, in an alcoholic family a direct action response may be the spouse leaving the alcoholic. Active coping strategies in an alcoholic family also include seeking counseling or therapy, and attending self-help groups (e.g., Al-Anon,

---

[3] **Morphogenesis** may be defined here as structural change within the family unit.

Adult Children of Alcoholics {ACOA}, AA). Active coping strategies are positive in nature since they tend to alter or attempt to change the stressful situation. Individuals that seek help through counseling or support groups inevitably may learn appropriate coping skills and behaviors that will not repeat the alcoholic family cycle of dysfunctional behavior.

Palliative coping strategies are emotive or cognitive responses to a troubled situation that attempt to reduce the individual's psychic pain. Since these responses are inward in nature, they do not alter the situation, but are intended to reduce the individual's psychic or emotional pain. A palliative coping strategy would be denial of the harmful or painful situation, or the use of alcohol or drugs to mask or sedate the psychic pain experienced by the individual. Both denial and alcohol or drug use are frequent palliative coping strategies in alcoholic families. But not only are denial and the use of alcohol and drugs palliative coping responses, they are also negative coping strategies which do not alter the painful situation but tend to prolong it since no active or constructive measures are taken to change the situation.

Another form of a palliative coping strategy on the part of the child within the alcoholic family is taking on parental responsibilities or becoming over-responsible. Taking on responsibility provides stability for the child within a dysfunctional family system. Children find ways to provide structure and consistency when not provided by the parents. In a healthy family, the child may exhibit "helping out Mom and Dad" behaviors. In the healthy family the child or children and parents are aware that the child is "helping out" rather than the child exchanging places with the parent on a permanent basis in terms of his/her responsibilities.

Therefore, in a dysfunctional family situation "the 'responsibility' is adopted by the child to cope with the disequilibrium or is advocated by the parent and accepted by the child."[79] Taking on responsibility as a child becomes an important part of identity formation. Furthermore, taking on adult responsibilities may have been influenced by both overt and covert variables. In order to give stability and consistency to his/her life, overtly the child took on the responsibilities as a coping strategy.

Covertly, the child may have found comfort in caring for the family's needs in that his/her identity was defined in the context of the relationship and affiliation with family members. However, the child was thrust into an adult role for which he/she was initially too young and unprepared for. Taking on adult responsibilities in order to find stability and consistency many times leads to controlling and rigid behaviors in adulthood. Table 6.3 illustrates the cycle of dysfunction within the alcoholic family with the consequences of either palliative or active coping strategies.

McCubbin and Patterson in their studies of families in crises contended that certain factors are beneficial to a family coping with a stressful situation. Coping resources that enable a healthy family to deal with and resolve stressful situations were identified by McCubbin and Patterson (1982) as: "(a) self-reliance and self-esteem, (b) family integration, (c) social support, (d) social action, and (e) collective group support."[80] These coping resources appear to be missing from most alcoholic family's repertoire or coping strategies.

It is evident that coping, whether overtly or covertly, is an active process that relies on family resources. Family resources enable the family members to deal with and mature due

Table 6.3

Children of Alcoholic Parents and the Paradigm of the Family Cycle of Dysfunction

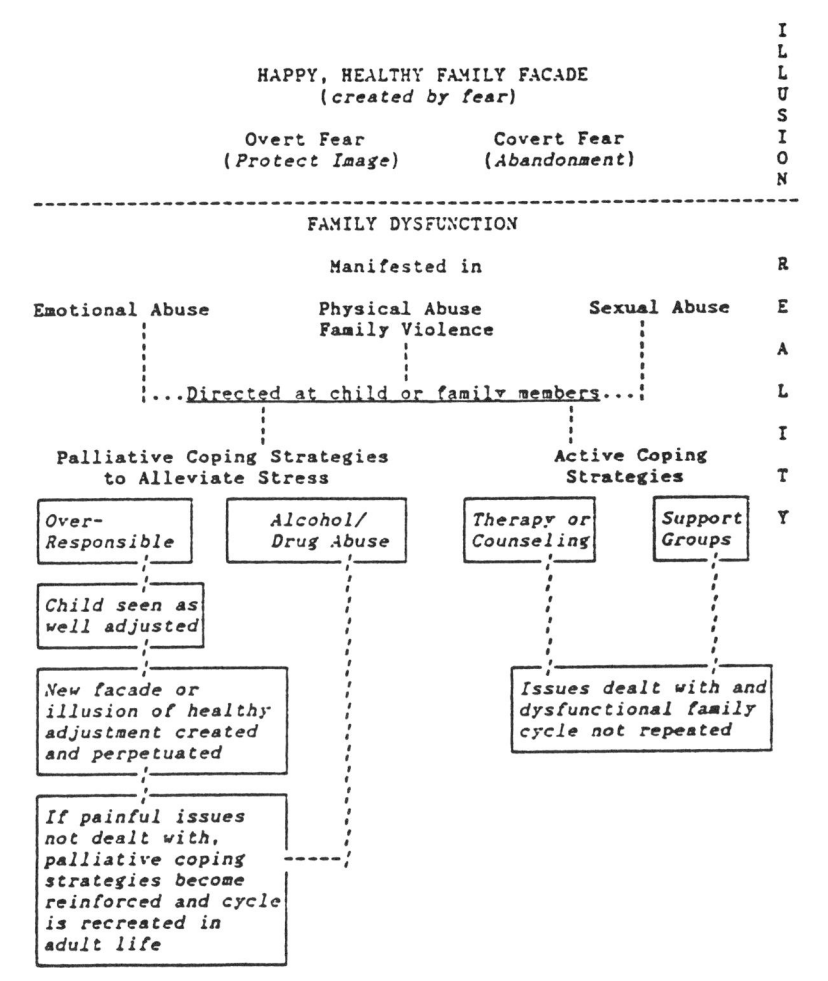

```
                                                              I
                                                              L
              HAPPY, HEALTHY FAMILY FACADE                    L
                    (created by fear)                         U
                                                              S
              Overt Fear          Covert Fear                 I
            (Protect Image)      (Abandonment)                O
                                                              N
-------------------------------------------------------------
                     FAMILY DYSFUNCTION
                       Manifested in                          R

 Emotional Abuse      Physical Abuse       Sexual Abuse       E
                      Family Violence
                                                              A
              ...Directed at child or family members...       L

                                                              I
   Palliative Coping Strategies         Active Coping
       to Alleviate Stress               Strategies           T

 ┌──────────┐  ┌──────────┐   ┌──────────┐  ┌──────────┐      Y
 │ Over-    │  │ Alcohol/ │   │Therapy or│  │ Support  │
 │Responsible│ │Drug Abuse│   │Counseling│  │ Groups   │
 └──────────┘  └──────────┘   └──────────┘  └──────────┘

 ┌──────────┐
 │Child seen as│
 │well adjusted│
 └──────────┘
                                ┌──────────────────────┐
 ┌──────────────┐                │ Issues dealt with and│
 │New facade or │                │ dysfunctional family │
 │illusion of healthy│           │ cycle not repeated   │
 │adjustment created│            └──────────────────────┘
 │and perpetuated│
 └──────────────┘

 ┌──────────────┐
 │If painful issues│
 │not dealt with, │
 │palliative coping│----
 │strategies become│
 │reinforced and cycle│
 │is recreated in │
 │adult life      │
 └──────────────┘
```

149

to the crisis situation, or conversely, reinforce the negative and dysfunctional coping strategies such as denial or alcohol and drug use. According to researchers, cohesion and adaptability are family resources that maintain the healthy functioning of the family during a crisis situation. Olson and McCubbin define family cohesion "as the emotional bonding that family members have toward one another and the degree of individual autonomy they experience."[81] Within the dimensions of emotional bonding, independence, family boundaries, friends, decision making, etc. family members can become either disengaged or enmeshed.

An example of a disengaged system is when family members have weak family affiliations, and high independence of family members is fostered. Any emotional bonding within an disengaged family system is seen as very low. An example of an enmeshed family system is when parental and child boundaries are blurred with no clear separation of parent/child responsibilities or roles. Emotional bonding is seen as very high, at times to the point of exclusion of a person's individuality. To achieve an optimum healthy level of cohesion, balance is necessary. Family members need to deal with and respond appropriately to crisis with support from other family members.

Adaptability within a family is defined by Olson and McCubbin "as the ability of a marital or family system to change its power structure, role relationships, and relationship rules in response to situational and development stress."[82] However, once the stress has been dealt with and alleviated, the family members within a healthy family unit resume their appropriate roles and relationships as parents, children and siblings. Dimensions of family adaptability range from chaotic to flexible to structured to rigid family patterns. Chaotic family patterns include dramatic rule and role changes, poor problem solving and either passive or aggressive assertiveness styles. Flexible family adaptability patterns include role sharing, good problem solving skills and some rule changes. Structured family patterns include some role sharing, few rule changes with consistent and predictable consequences with control of family being maintained by one leader. A rigid family system is depicted by rigid rules and roles, strict enforcement with an overly strict discipline model. As in family cohesion, balanced levels of family adaptability distinguish functional families from unhealthy or dysfunctional families.

Olson and McCubbin postulated that balance is critical and that problematic families often function at either of the extremes leading to either chaos or no change which results in rigidity. It was also suggested that more functional or balanced families develop and maintain a larger repertoire of behaviors when faced with crisis situations as opposed to dysfunctional families which tend to function on rigid dimensions.

Kritsberg views the alcoholic family and the healthy family at opposite ends of a continuum. The alcoholic family has rigid rules and roles, a keeper of family secrets, resisting outsiders from entering the family system, unclear personal boundaries, and with no personal privacy. Within the alcoholic family, family members are rarely free to leave the system. And although a loyalty seems to exist within this family, it is a facade, with no unity among members.[83]

In contrast, Kritsberg views the healthy family with flexible rules and roles, no family secrets, maintaining a sense of humor, and welcoming of outsiders to the family. The healthy family maintains privacy for all its members and allows members to develop a sense of self. Conflict among family members is allowed and resolved. Family change is seen as continual growth with a sense of wholeness to the unit. According to these dimensions, the alcoholic family is seen as enmeshed with unclear or blurred boundaries and fluctuating between the chaotic and rigid family patterns.

As a result of stress encountered in the alcoholic family, the child may encounter demands by parents and/or siblings which are inappropriate for the child's age.[84] For example, rather than the parent having primary responsibility over the care of the children, in the alcoholic family this responsibility may be relegated to an older sibling. Therefore, the sibling in his/her behavior may be the "parent" of the younger siblings, whereas the rigid and often arbitrary rules are set by the alcoholic parent acting in the parental role. Role distortions, therefore, interfere with the proper channeling of the child's role learning abilities.[85]

In fact, the manifestation of inconsistent, unpredictable behavior on the part of the parents tends to discourage the child's problem solving abilities due to the inability of the child to predict parental actions. Since, at various times, the child may be treated like a parent, spouse or child, the child may experience tension and conflict when faced with role shifting. What may ensue from trying to deal with unpredictable and conflicting models of parental behavior is a negative coping style on the part of the child. Ineffectual parenting skills and disrupted family patterns (as frequently observed in alcoholic families) are significantly related to a youth's suicidal behavior or self-destructive coping strategies.[86,87]

Seixas and Youcha contended that due to the stress experienced by the children of alcoholic parents, youngsters develop survival skills and "adjust no matter how unstable or difficult their lives may be."[88] One of the ways this negative coping style may manifest itself is as low self-esteem with feelings of inferiority or disparagement. Cleveland and Longaker define disparagement as an "habitual choice of extreme devaluation of a pattern for coping with problems of an intrapsychic or interpersonal nature."[89] In other words, the child within the alcoholic family system due to the constant stress, role shifting and unpredictable behavior among family members may resort to negative coping strategies and subsequent neurotic behavior.

Researchers have shown that stress originating within the family is seen as disorganizing and demoralizing since the stress causes a disturbance in role patterns. Whereas external family stress events such as wars, natural disasters, etc., tend to bring the family together, internal stresses tend to disorganize and breakdown the family.

SUMMARY

Parental alcoholism predisposes the child to behavioral and emotional problems, as well as alcoholism. Whether genetically predisposed or a learned behavior, alcoholism continues to be the highest among children of alcoholic parents. High levels of stress and inconsistent behavior on the part of the parents, ultimately force the child to deal with the stress either through appropriate or inappropriate coping methods. Coping methods manifest themselves either in palliative or negative coping styles such as becoming over-responsible, or alcohol use and abuse; or in active or positive coping strategies such as in seeking counseling or attending self-help groups (e.g., Al-Anon, AA, etc.). The family cycle of dysfunction has a greater chance of repeating the dysfunctional system if the child resorts to palliative coping strategies to alleviate stress. If measures are taken to alleviate stress through active methods such as seeking either professional or self-help support services, the dysfunctional system is hopefully averted.

REFERENCES

1. Ackerman, R. J., **Children of Alcoholics**, 2nd Ed., Learning Publications, Holmes Beach, Florida, 1979.
2. Bosma, W., Alcoholism and teenagers, **Maryland State Medical Journal**, 24(6), 62, 1975.
3. Drew, L. R. H., Moon, J. R., and Buchanan, F. H., **Alcoholism: A Handbook**, Heinemann Heath Books, Melbourne, Australia, 1974.
4. Gravitz, H. L. and Bowden, J. D., Therapeutic issues of adult children of alcoholics, **Alcohol Health and Research World**, 8(4), 25, 1984.
5. Johnson, J. L., Sher, K. J., and Rolf, J. E., Models of vulnerability to psychopathology in children of alcoholics, **Alcohol Health and Research World**, 15(1), 33, 1991.
6. Lawson, G., Peterson, J. S., and Lawson, A., **Alcoholism and the Family**, Aspen, Rockville, Maryland, 1983.
7. McKenna, R. and Pickens, R., Personality characteristics of alcoholic children of alcoholics, **Journal of Studies on Alcohol**, 44(4), 688, 1981.
8. Moser, J., **Prevention of Alcohol-Related Problems: An International Review of Preventive Measures, Policies and Programmes**, Alcoholism and Drug Addiction Research Foundation, Toronto, Canada, 1980.
9. Pilat, J. M. and Jones, J. W., Identification of children of alcoholics: Two empirical studies, **Alcohol Health and Research World**, 9(2), 27, 1984/85.
10. Russell, M., Henderson, C., and Blume, S. B., **Children of Alcoholics: A Review of the Literature**, Children of Alcoholics Foundation, New York, 1985.

11. Drew, **Alcoholism**, 1974.
12. Bosma, **Alcoholism**, 1975.
13. Gravitz, **Therapeutic**, 1984.
14. Hawkins, J. D., Lishner, D. M., Catalano, R. F., and Howard, M. O., Childhood predictors of adolescent substance abuse: Toward an empirically grounded theory, **Journal of Children in Contemporary Society, 8**(1), 11, 1986.
15. Lawson, **Alcoholism**, 1983.
16. Moser, **Prevention**, 1980.
17. Pilat, **Identification**, 1984/85.
18. Searles, J. S., The role of genetics in the pathogenesis of alcoholism, **Journal of Abnormal Psychology, 97**, 153, 1988.
19. Beardslee, W. R., Son, L., and Vaillant, G. E., Exposure to parental alcoholism during childhood and outcome in adulthood: A prospective longitudinal study, **British Journal of Psychiatry, 149**, 584, 1986.
20. Lisansky, E. S., Alcoholism in women: Social and psychological concomitants, **Quarterly Journal Studies on Alcoholism, 18**, 588, 1957.
21. Mulford, H. A., Women and men - problem drinking: Sex differences in patients served by Iowa's Community Alcoholism Centers, **Journal of Studies on Alcohol, 38**, 1627, 1977.
22. Sherfey, M. J., Psychopathy and character structure in chronic alcoholism, in **Etiology of Chronic Alcoholism**, Diethelm, O., Ed., Charles C. Thomas, Springfield, Illinois,1955.
23. Corrigan, E. M., **Alcoholic Women in Treatment**, Oxford University Press, New York, 1980.
24. O'Connor, S., Hesselbrock, V., and Bauer, L., The nervous system and the predisposition to alcoholism, **Alcohol Health and Research World, 14**, 90, 1990.
25. McCaul, M. E., Svikis, D. S., Turkkan, J. S., Bigelow, G. E., and Cromwell, C. C., Degree of familial alcoholism: Effects on substance abuse by college males, in **Problems**

of Drug Dependence 1989. Proceedings of the 51st Annual Scientific Meeting, Research Monograph #95, Harris, L. W., Ed., National Institute on Drug Abuse, Rockville, Maryland, 1989.

26. Hrubec, Z. and Omenn, G., Evidence of genetic predisposition to alcoholic cirrhosis and psychosis: Twin concordances for alcoholism and its biological end points by zygosity among male veterans, **Alcoholism: Clinical and Experimental Research**, 5, 207, 1981.

27. Plomin, R., Defries, J., and McClearn, G. E., **Behavioral Genetics: A Primer**, W. H. Freeman, New York, 1990.

28. Kaij, L., **Studies on the Etiology and Sequels of Abuse of Alcohol**, Department of Psychiatry, University of Lund, Lund, Sweden, 1960.

29. Bohman, M., Cloninger, C. R., Von Knorring, A. L., and Sigvardsson, S., An adoption study of somatoform disorders: III. Cross-fostering analysis and genetic relationship to alcoholism and criminality, **Archives of General Psychiatry**, 41(9), 872, 1984.

30. Cadoret, R. J., Cain, C. A., and Grove, W. M., Development of alcoholism in adoptees raised apart from alcoholic biologic relatives, **Archives of General Psychiatry**, 37(5), 561, 1980.

31. Cloninger, C. R, Bohman, M., and Sigvardsson, S., Inheritance of alcohol abuse: Cross fostering analysis of adopted men, **Archives of General Psychiatry**, 38(8), 861, 1981.

32. Goodwin, D. W., Schulsinger, F., Hermanson, L., Guze, S. B., and Winokur, G., Alcohol problems in adoptees raised apart from alcoholic biological parents, **Archives of General Psychiatry**, 28, 238, 1973.

33. Beckman, L. J., Women alcoholics: A review of social and psychological studies, **Quarterly Journal of Studies on Alcohol**, 36,

797, 1975.

34. Brown, G. and Harris, I., **The Social Origins of Depression**, Tavistock, London, 1978.

35. Corrigan, **Alcoholic**, 1980.

36. Wilson, C., The family, in **Women and Alcohol**, Camberwell Council on Alcoholism, Eds., Tavistock, London, 1980.

37. Cork, R. M., **The Forgotten Children**, Alcoholism and Drug Addiction Research Foundation, 1969.

38. Ackerman, **Children**, 1979.

39. Gravitz, **Therapeutic**, 1984.

40. Lawson, **Alcoholism**, 1983.

41. Kammeier, M. L., Adolescents from families with and without alcohol problems, **Quarterly Journal of Studies in Alcoholism, 32**, 364, 1971.

42. Jacob, R., Favorini, A., Meisel, S. S., and Anderson, C. M., The alcoholic's spouse, children and family interactions: Substantive findings and methodological issues, **Journal of Studies on Alcohol, 39**(7), 1231, 1978.

43. Cermak, R. L., Children of alcoholics and the case for a new diagnostic category of co-dependence, **Alcohol Health and Research World, 84**(4), 38, 1984.

44. McKenna, **Personality**, 1981.

45. West, M. O. and Prinz, R. J., Parental alcoholism and childhood psychopathology, **Psychological Bulletin, 102**(2), 204, 1987.

46. Achenbach, T. M., Internalizing disorders: Subtyping based on parental questionnaire, in **Needs and Prospects of Child and Adolescent Psychiatry**, Schmidt, M. H. and Remschmidt, H., Eds., Hogrefe and Huber, Toronto, 1989.

47. Johnson, **Models**, 1991.

48. Beardslee, **Exposure**, 1986.

49. Russell, Children, 1985.

50. Robins, L. H., Conduct disorder, **Journal of Child Psychology and Psychiatry, 31**(1), 193, 1991.

51. Cloninger, **Inheritance**, 1981.
52. Noyes, R. Jr., Clancy, J., and Crowe, R., The familial prevalence of anxiety neurosis, **Archives of General Psychiatry, 37**, 173, 1978.
53. West, **Parental**, 1987.
54. Clair, D. and Genest, M., Variables associated with the adjustment of offspring of alcoholic fathers, **Journal of Studies of Alcohol, 46**(4), 345, 1981.
55. Glenn, S. W. and Parsons, O. A., Alcohol abuse and familial alcoholism: Psychosocial correlates in men and women, **Journal of Studies on Alcohol, 50**(2), 116, 1989.
56. Parker, D. A. and Harford, T. C., Alcohol-related problems marital disruption and depressive symptoms among adult children of alcohol abusers in the United States, **Journal of Studies in Alcohol, 49**(4), 306, 1988.
57. Christopoulos, C., Cohn, D. A., Shaw, D. S., Joyce, S., Sullivan-Hanson, J., Kraft, S., and Emery, R. E., Children of abused women: I. Adjustment at time of shelter residence, **Journal of Marriage and the Family, 49**, 611, 1987.
58. Emery, R. E., Family violence, **American Psychologist, 44**(2), 321, 1989.
59. Hughes, H. M. and Barad, S., Psychological functioning of children in a battered women's shelter: A preliminary investigation, **American Journal of Orthopsychiatry, 53**, 525, 1983.
60. Kalmuss, D., The intergenerational transmission of marital aggression, **Journal of Marriage and the Family, 47**, 11, 1984.
61. Rosenberg, M. S., New directions for research on the psychological maltreatment of children, **American Psychologist, 42**, 166, 1987.
62. Figley, C. R., Catastrophes: An overview of family reactions, in **Stress and the Family**, Figley, C. R. and McCubbin, H. I,

Eds., Brunner/Mazel, New York, 1983.

63. Frederick, C., Effects of natural versus human-induced violence upon the victim, **Evaluation and Change, Special Issue, 71**, 1980.

64. Putnam, R. W., Post, R. M., and Guroff, J. J., One Hundred Cases of Multiple Personality Disorder, paper presented at the annual meeting of the American Psychiatric Association, Los Angeles, California, May, 1984.

65. Bell, N. W., Extended family relations of disturbed and well families, in **The Psychosocial Interior of the Family**, 3rd Ed., Handel, G., Ed., Aldine, New York, 1985, p. 159.

66. Deutsch, C., **Broken Bottles, Broken Dreams: Understanding and Helping the Children of Alcoholics**, Teachers College Press, New York, 1982.

67. Caplan, G., The family as a support system, in **Family Stress, Coping and Social Support**, Cauble, A. E. and Patterson, J. M., Eds., Charles C. Thomas, Springfield, Illinois, 1982.

68. Lee, G. R., **Family Structure and Interaction: A Comparative Analysis**, 2nd Ed., University of Minnesota Press, Minneapolis, Minnesota, 1982.

69. Lazarus, R., **Psychological Stress and the Coping Process**, McGraw Hill, New York, 1966.

70. McCubbin, H. I., Cauble, A. E., and Patterson, J. M., Eds., **Family Stress, Coping, and Social Support**, Charles C. Thomas, Springfield, Illinois, 1982.

71. Erikson, E., **Childhood and Society**, Norton, New York, 1963.

72. McCubbin, **Family**, 1982, p. xii.

73. Duncan, D., Family stress and the initiation of adolescent drug abuse: A retrospective study, **Corrective and Social Psychiatry, 24**(3), 111, 1978.

74. Cermak, **Children**, 1984.

75. Kaufman, E., The family of the alcoholic parent, **Psychosomatics, 27**(5), 347, 1986.
76. Brown, S., **Treating Adult Children of Alcoholics: A Developmental Perspective**, John Wiley and Sons, New York, 1988.
77. McCubbin, **Family**, 1982.
78. Lazarus, **Psychological**, 1966.
79. Brown, **Treating**, 1988, p. 176.
80. McCubbin, H. I. and Patterson, J. M., Family adaptation to crises, in **Family Stress, Coping, and Social Support**, McCubbin, H. I., Cauble, A. E., and Patterson, J. M., Eds., Charles C. Thomas, Springfield, Illinois, 1982, p. 37.
81. Olson, D. H. and McCubbin, H. I., Circumplex model of marital and family systems. V: Application to family stress and crisis interventions, in **Family Stress Coping, and Social Support**, McCubbin, H. I., Cauble, A. E., and Patterson, J. M., Eds., Charles C. Thomas, Springfield, Illinois, 1982, p. 49.
82. Olson, **Circumplex**, 1982, p. 51.
83. Kritsberg, W., **Adult Children of Alcoholics Syndrome**, Bantam, New York, 1988.
84. Jacob, **Alcoholic's Spouse**, 1978.
85. Lidz, T., **The Origins and Treatment of Schizophrenic Disorders**, Basic Books, New York, 1973.
86. Patros, P. G. and Shamoo, T. K., **Depression and Suicide in Children and Adolescents: Prevention, Intervention and Postvention**, Allyn and Bacon, Boston, 1989.
87. Pfeffer, C. R., The family system of suicidal children, **American Journal of Psychotherapy, 35**, 330, 1981.
88. Seixas, J. S. and Youcha, G., **Children of Alcoholism: A Survivor's Manual**, Crown, New York, 1985.
89. Cleveland, E. J. and Longaker, W. D., Neurotic patterns in the family, in **The Psychosocial Interior of the Family**, 3rd Ed., Aldine, New York, 1985.

Chapter 7

ALCOHOL AND HOMELESSNESS

In 1990, the United States Bureau of the Census revealed that the recent number of homeless individuals is in the range of 228,372. This figure is comprised of two components. First, 178,638 individuals were counted in emergency shelters, and second, 49,734 individuals were counted in "visible, street locations". "Visible, street locations" refers to individuals living outside and apart from shelters or centers.[1] Since this is an elusive population in which to gather statistics, the most recent figure may be a gross underestimate of the prevalence of homelessness in this nation. The United States Department of Housing and Urban Development has estimated the number of homeless individuals to be approximately 250,000. However, the Washington, D. C. based Community for Creative Non-Violence has assessed the figure to be closer to 3 million.[2]

Homelessness is a growing problem in the United States and the rate has more than tripled since 1979.[3,4] Furthermore, between 20 and 45 percent of the homeless population is believed to have alcohol-related problems.[5] Studies have repeatedly indicated that alcohol abuse is widespread among the homeless population and often has played a key role in becoming homeless. In a study conducted with homeless adults in Los Angeles, findings indicated that 62.9 percent of the inner-city homeless met the criteria for either alcohol abuse or dependence.[6,7]

In an article concerning homelessness, Hilfiker stated that "the tragedy of substance abuse among the very poor cannot be underestimated, and the treatment of coexisting health problems is enormously complicated."[8] Hilfiker also stated that the scarcity of or inaccessibility to health care, including mental health and substance abuse services, as well as unsanitary living conditions, contributes to the overwhelming problems experienced by the homeless.

Although initially the homeless person was considered to be the skid row bum, the homeless population today includes women, adolescents, the elderly, and families. The heterogenous group that comprises the homeless population, faces the multiple risks of poverty, physical disability, mental illness, malnutrition, dehydration, and polydrug use. It is well documented that alcohol abuse without any other pre-existing physical or mental condition causes a wide variety of digestive, endocrinological, neurological, circulatory, psychiatric, and nutritional disorders. When adding homelessness to alcohol abuse, the debilitating results of both are compounded.

Wright and colleagues have cited that homeless alcohol abusers can be expected to have both the diseases and disorders characteristic of both alcohol abusers and homeless in general. Homeless alcohol abusing males, when compared to homeless men in general, were at a higher than average risk for experiencing trauma, as well as, developing gastrointestinal disorders, cardiovascular disorders, lung and liver diseases, hypertension, and neurological impairments. Overall, alcohol abusing homeless individuals were found to be much sicker than average when compared with non-alcohol abusing individuals.[10]

A study conducted in 16 U. S. cities with over 11,000 homeless men and women who were identified as problem drinkers revealed that alcohol abusing homeless adults were "four to seven times as likely to suffer from liver disease, twice as likely to suffer serious traumas, two to three times as likely to be disabled by seizure disorders or other neurological impairments, and also twice as likely to present with various nutritional deficiencies (predominantly malnutrition and dehydration)."[11] Hypertension, chronic obstructive pulmonary disease, gastrointestinal disorders and arterial diseases were 50 percent more common among alcohol abusing homeless adults than among non-alcohol abusing homeless individuals. Since many heavy alcohol drinkers also are heavy smokers, homeless alcohol abusing adults are also at a very high risk of lung disorders.

Based on the findings of this study, alcohol abuse was characteristic of 40 to 50 percent of homeless men and approximately 10 to 20 percent of homeless women. In addition to suffering physical disorders at a higher rate than non-alcohol abusing homeless adults, alcohol abusing homeless individuals also had higher rates of drug abuse and mental illness.[12] Koegel & Burnam indicated that the presence of psychiatric disorders (e.g., affective disorders, panic disorder, etc.) as defined by the **DSM-III** among alcohol abusing homeless adults appeared to be higher overall when compared with non-alcohol abusing homeless individuals. Furthermore, a significant difference was found pertaining to antisocial personality and drug abuse or dependence disorders among homeless individuals with an alcohol diagnosis when compared with homeless adults with no alcohol diagnosis. Table 7.1 (adapted from Koegel and Burnam [14]) illustrates this difference.

In addition to the **DSM-III** defined disorders experienced by homeless individuals with an alcohol diagnosis, this group was also found to be undergoing more psychological distress than the "no alcohol diagnosis" group. The issue of homeless alcoholics experiencing greater emotional distress was also supported by the Baltimore Homeless Study conducted in 1986 with 162 homeless men and women. This study also suggested linkages between

Table 7.1

Presence of Lifetime DSM-III Disorders Among Homeless Persons

	Alcohol Diagnosis	No Alcohol Diagnosis
Antisocial personality**	29.7%	6.1%
Drug abuse or dependence**	39.0	17.5

** $p < .001$

alcoholism and psychiatric disorders among the homeless. Of interest in the Fischer and Breakey study is the fact that approximately one-half of the alcoholics believed that drinking was a major contributing factor to their becoming homeless.[15]

A study conducted by Shandler & Shipley with homeless adults in Philadelphia corroborated the previous findings of alcohol-abusing individuals experiencing a higher rate of physical and psychiatric disorders. In the winter of 1985-1986, homeless people were required to go to an emergency shelter when the windchill factor dropped to 10 degrees. Of the 162 alcohol abusing homeless individuals that came to the shelter, 95 percent were males, and 84 percent had measurable blood alcohol levels (BALs) ranging up to .38 percent, with the median BAL being .14 percent. One hundred and eight or 67 percent of the 162 homeless individuals completed a physical examination. The following are the results of this medical evaluation: 44 percent of the alcohol abusing homeless individuals had liver problems, 29 percent suffered from fractures, abrasions and other traumas, 27 percent had respiratory problems, 18 percent were malnourished, 10 percent were diagnosed with gastritis, 26 percent had a history of seizures, and 25 percent had significant psychiatric problems. Based on the results of this medical examination, 22 percent required hospitalization for detoxification and 41 percent were placed in a nonhospital detox unit. The authors concluded that over 75 percent of the homeless individuals with an alcohol diagnosis had serious physical problems and a serious problem with alcohol.[16]

In a more recent study conducted by Breakey and colleagues, the Baltimore Homeless Study with 528 homeless individuals, researchers found the most frequently cited health problems included mouth and dental problems, gynecologic, dermatologic, cardiovascular, musculoskeletal, respiratory, and neurological disorders, as well as anemia, and sexually transmitted diseases. The primary use of alcohol in this population was observed in 85 percent of the males and 67 percent of the females.[17]

The difference between homeless individuals who congregated in shelters and homeless who lived and slept outdoors was examined by Gelberg and Linn. In their study, Gelberg and Linn found that homeless who utilized shelters were less likely to have experienced an injury or trauma, less likely to smoke cigarettes and to use drugs. In comparison, the outdoor group reported more vomiting or diarrhea and drinking alcohol on a daily basis. The outdoor group was also found to have elevated liver enzymes, elevated mean corpuscular hemoglobin concentrations, elevated globulin levels, high lactate dehydrogenase levels, and low serum urea nitrogen levels. Overall, the outdoor group had the most physical health problems as compared with individuals using shelters. Gelberg and Linn concluded that the most worrisome finding of this study was the fact that persons living primarily outdoors were more likely to report alcoholic behavior and to have physical complications related to the alcohol problem. But despite the fact that the outdoor group clearly needed health and substance abuse services, this assistance was not available.[18]

SUMMARY

Alcohol abuse and dependence among the homeless population has been linked with a wide array of documented physical and psychiatric disorders. Among the physical disorders noted are hypertension, chronic obstructive pulmonary disease, gastrointestinal disorders, arterial diseases, anemia, sexually transmitted diseases, and neurological impairments. Psychiatric disturbances in the form of affective disorders, panic disorder, or antisocial personality disorders were also documented.

Researchers have also identified that homeless adults with alcohol problems were homeless for a longer period of time and appeared more transient than nonalcoholic homeless individuals.[19] Overall, the most frequent disorders cited among the homeless population were those connected with substance abuse, primarily alcohol.[20]

REFERENCES

1. United States Bureau of the Census, **Homeless Statistics**, U. S. Department of Commerce, Washington, D. C., 1990.

2. Lubran, B. G., Alcohol-related problems among the homeless, **Alcohol Health and Research World, D11**(3), 4, 1987.

3. Gelberg, L. and Linn, L. S., Assessing the physical health of homeless adults, **The Journal of the American Medical Association, 262**, 1973, 1989.

4. Herman, M., Galanter, M., and Lifshutz, H., Combined substance abuse and psychiatric disorders in homeless and domiciled patients, **American Journal of Drug and Alcohol Abuse, 17**, 415, 1991.

5. Lubran, **Alcohol**, 1987.

6. Koegel, P. and Burnam, M. A., Traditional and nontraditional homeless alcoholics, **Alcohol Health and Research World, 11**(3), 28, 1987.

7. Pinkney, D. S., Looking at how people 'drop through the cracks': APA (American Psychiatric Association) panel focuses on woes of the homeless, **American Medical News, 33**, 3, July 20, 1990.

8. Hilfiker, D., Are we comfortable with homelessness? (Commentary/caring for the poor), **The Journal of the American Medical Association, 262**, 1375, 1989.

9. Wright, J. D., Knight, J. W., Weber-Burdin, E., and Lam, J., Ailments and alcohol: Health status among the drinking homeless, **Alcohol Health and Research World, 11**(3), 22, 1987.

10. Wright, J. D., Rossi, P. H., Knight, J. W., Weber-Burdin, E., Tessler, R. C., Stewart, C. E., Geronimo, M., and Lam, J., Health and homelessness: An analysis of the health status of a sample of homeless people receiving care through the Department of Community Medicine, St. Vincent's Hospital and Medical Center of New York City: 1969-1984, Social and Demographic Research Institute, Amherst, Massachusetts, 1985.

11. Wright, **Ailments**, 1987, p. 24.

12. Wright, **Ailments**, 1987.

13. Koegel, **Traditional**, 1987.

14. Koegel, **Traditional**, 1987.

15. Fischer, P. J. and Breakey, W. R., Profile of the Baltimore homeless with alcohol problems, **Alcohol Health and Research World, 11**(3), 36, 1987.

16. Shandler, I. W. and Shipley, T. E. Jr., New focus for an old problem: Philadelphia's

response to homelessness, **Alcohol Health and Research World, 11**(3), 54, 1987.

17. Breakey, W. R., Fischer, P. J., Kramer, M., Nestadt, F., Romanoski, A. J., Ross, A., Royall, R. M., and Stine, O. C., Health and mental health problems of homeless men and women in Baltimore, **The Journal of the American Medical Association, 262**, 1352, 1989.

18. Gelberg, **Assessing**, 1989.

19. Roth, D. and Bean, J., Alcohol problems and homelessness: Findings from the Ohio study, **Alcohol Health and Research World, 10**(2), 14, 1985/86.

20. Breakey, **Health**, 1989.

Chapter 8

ALCOHOL ASSESSMENT TOOLS

I. ALCOHOL USE EVALUATIONS

Assessing the extent of alcohol involvement is crucial in determining the most potentially successful treatment approach. A number of tools have been developed to determine whether an individual has a drinking problem. One of the easiest tools is in the form of a simple questionnaire. With this questionnaire, a person in his/her own privacy answers "yes" or "no" to a series of questions pertaining to drinking. The following is a sample questionnaire form.

A. ALCOHOL USE QUESTIONNAIRE

Answer "yes" or "no" to the following questions. Answer as honestly as you can.

1. Do you drink alcohol to relieve stress or emotional discomfort?
2. Do you drink alcohol despite your family's request to stop?
3. Do you drink alcohol in order to feel more outgoing, brave, self-confident, or assertive?
4. Have you experienced blackouts or gaps in memory after an episode of drinking?
5. Do you become defensive or upset if someone comments on your drinking?
6. Do you crave a drink at certain times of the day?
7. Has your job performance been affected by your drinking? For example, have you called in sick or late after a night of drinking.
8. Do you drink alone?
9. Have you ever been hospitalized due to drinking?
10. Do you feel regret after drinking?
11. Have you ever driven an automobile

despite the fact that you had been drinking and felt out of control?
12. Are you experiencing financial problems due to your drinking?
13. Are you experiencing marital and family problems due to your drinking?
14. Has your physical health been affected as a result of drinking?
15. Have you ever been stopped or arrested for drinking and driving?
16. Do you feel nervous or agitated when you know you can't have a drink?

If you answered YES to any of the questions, you may have a problem with drinking.

If you answered YES to two or more questions, you may wish to speak with your doctor, alcohol specialist or counselor t o learn more about alcohol abuse and treatments available.

If the person determines that he/she may in fact have a problem with alcohol, the person should seek guidance from an individual skilled in alcohol abuse counseling. Before the alcohol abuse counselor may recommend any treatment plan, the counselor needs to complete a comprehensive history of the individual. This comprehensive history is also known as a Psychosocial Evaluation. The Psychosocial Evaluation is a series of questions that addresses family history, alcohol/drug history, and a mental status exam. The following is an example of a Psychosocial Evaluation together with sample questions that may be asked of the individual during the interview process:

B. PSYCHOSOCIAL EVALUATION

Presenting Problem:
After the counselor has obtained all the pertinent demographic data, such as name,

address, place of employment, etc., the counselor may ask the client the following questions:

-Can you tell me what brings you here today?
-Can you tell me how long this (the problem) has been happening?
-Approximately when did this problem start?

Previous Treatment:

After determining the reason why the individual is seeking counseling, it is important to find out if the person has received previous help. Often an individual goes into counseling for a number of reasons, such as:

(1) The person is experiencing a difficult situation and is serious in making changes in his/her life. This person is ready to look at some possibly painful issues in his/her life, and with the assistance of a trained counselor determine the appropriate course of action.

(2) This person is looking for a quick and easy solution to ease the pain a problem may be causing, but it is unlikely the person will stay in counseling long-term to make any lasting changes. Counseling is often a painful process. Unless the person is ready to work hard and make some important changes, the symptoms may be temporarily eased, but the problem will not go away and eventually resurface.

Either Person #1 or Person #2 may have been in counseling before. Person #1 may have had success in counseling in the past and is
ready to work on unresolved issues. Person #2 may be "therapy shopping" or "counseling hopping". This person may be looking for the "quick fix". This type of client unfortunately is under the impression that an easing of emotional pain is the same as resolving the problem. Either Person #1 or Person #2 may have been in counseling before but for entirely different reasons. The astute counselor will be able to deduce which course

of treatment is most appropriate through the following series of questions:
- Have you ever been in counseling before?
- For how long?
- Was this for the same problem?
- Do you feel you benefitted from this counseling?
- How did you benefit? or Why do you think you did not benefit from counseling?
- Were you prescribed medications? If yes, what are the medications and for what reason.
- Are you presently on medication? If yes, what is the medication and for what reason are you taking it? Dosage?
- Is there anything in particular you are looking for from counseling? Please be specific, if you can.

Personal History and Family History:

Before the counselor can begin to focus on the individual before him/her, it is important to gain an understanding of the person's family history. Within this family context, it is easier to understand certain behaviors, attitudes, beliefs, and values of the client. How the family has impacted upon, and/or continues to impact on the client will enable the counselor to comprehend the client's perceptual framework and problem solving abilities and behaviors.

Mother:
- How old is your mother?
- How is her health?
- Can you describe your relationship with your mother when you were growing up?
- Tell me about your relationship with your mother now?
- Did you mother drink alcohol? If yes, Can you tell me how much, on what occasions?
- Did she ever get drunk? If yes, what was her behavior like when she did get drunk?
- To your knowledge, did your mother ever use drugs?
- Did your mother use or is presently on prescribed drugs? For what reason?

Father:
- Same questions as for Mother.

Siblings:
- Do you have any brothers or sisters?
- What are their ages?
- To your knowledge do your brothers/sisters have any problems with alcohol or drugs?
- Is there any history of suicide attempts, depression or emotional problems in your family?
- Tell me about your relationship when you were growing up.
- How is your relationship now?
- How often do you see any of your family members?

Grandparents/Aunts/Uncles:
- Tell me about your grandmother, grandfather, aunt(s), uncle(s), etc.
- Is there any history of psychiatric or emotional problems, or alcohol/drug use or abuse to your knowledge?

General Family Questions:
- Has there been any physical abuse in your family? Can you tell me about it?
- Has there been any emotional abuse? Can you describe that to me?
- Has there been any sexual abuse? (This is the easiest question to say "no" to for various reasons: no memory or recollection of it (blocking), denial that it ever happened because of the trauma, or unable to confide in therapist yet. Accept the "no" answer. However, do not dismiss it completely.

Marital Status:
- Have you ever been married?
- How long have you been married?
- Is this your first marriage?
- If the client is living with someone, how long?
- How did you meet your spouse, significant other?
- What attracted you to him/her?
- Do you have any children?
- What are the children's ages?

-Describe your relationship with your children.

-How do you handle stressful situations with your children? What do you do when you get angry or upset with them?

-How do you handle stressful situations with your spouse/significant other?

Educational and Vocational History:

The client's experiences and history pertaining to education and career choices is an integral part of the comprehensive psychosocial evaluation. Data gathering pertaining to education and job history enables the counselor to understand how the individual gets along or interacts with people outside of the family network.

-What is the last grade you completed?

-Did you enjoy school? How were your grades?

-What kind of student were you?

-How did you get along with the other students? teachers?

-What were your favorite activities? least favorite?

-Tell me about your first job.

-Tell me about your job now. Where are you working? How long?

-Do you enjoy your work?

-How do you get along with your co-workers, supervisors, etc.?

If the individual's presenting problem is job and/or alcohol-related, the following questions need to be addressed related to job performance:

-Do you have frequent absences from work?

-What excuse do you frequently use when calling out?

-Are you frequently absent on Mondays or Fridays?

-Do you seem to have higher absences for gastritis, flu, etc. then other employees?

-Do your absences follow a pattern?

-Are you frequently late getting to work on time?

-Have you experienced any accidents on the job?
-Do you have difficulty concentrating at work?
-Do you make frequent mistakes while at work?
-Does work seem to take greater effort or tasks take longer to complete?
-Have you experienced a drop in work quality or work quantity?
-Are co-workers complaining about you?
-Have you had complaints from your supervisor? For what?
-Do you feel physically ill while at work?
-Do you drink while at lunch? How much? How often? How does drinking at lunch affect your work performance?
-How would your supervisor or co-worker answer the last question?
-Have you been given warnings regarding the quality or quantity of work?

Military History:

One area of questioning that is frequently overlooked when gathering data is the person's military history. Military history is particularly important if the person has been involved in a military action or active combat. The person's military experiences may have resulted in post-traumatic stress disorder. Survivors of combat or aversive military actions frequently self-medicate disturbing memories and thoughts through the use of alcohol. Very often the individual's first encounter with alcohol use and abuse is in the military. Therefore, it is important that the counselor ask the individual the following questions:

-Tell me about your military experiences.
-What branch of service were you in?
-How old were you when you joined?
-Were you involved in any military combat or aggressive action?
-Were you hurt while serving in the military?

176 ALCOHOL ASSESSMENT TOOLS

-Did you witness anyone hurt while in the military?
-How did your family or friends respond to or treat you when you returned?
-Do you feel that the military experience has changed you?
-How? Please be specific.
-Did you drink alcohol and/or take drugs to deal with the stress? How much? How often?

Legal History:

Obtaining information pertaining to legal history is especially important in determining the extent of the problems caused by alcohol abuse. The accuracy of this information is usually easier to get if the person has been referred for alcohol counseling due to drinking and driving, or criminal activity due to alcohol involvement. The best source of obtaining this information is through the probation officer and/or attorney.

-Have you ever been arrested?
-If yes, Please tell me about it. What were you arrested for?
-When? What was the outcome (jail, probation, fine, etc.)?
-Have you ever been arrested for drinking and driving? If yes, when? Why were you pulled over? What was your blood alcohol level (BAL)? (.10 is legal intoxication).
-What was the outcome? Are you on probation? Who is your probation officer? How often do you report to him/her?

Alcohol/Drug History:

Questions pertaining to alcohol/drug history are important to ask even if the "presenting problem" may not be alcohol related. Alcohol/drug history provides clues as to how the person copes with stress or relationships. It also provides clues as to how active alcohol/drug abuse/dependence may be impacting on the presenting problem; e.g., "I'm here because I'm having a rough time at work. My supervisor is on my back." This problem may be due to alcohol/drug related

issues.
Alcohol:
-How old were you when you had your first drink?
-Did you start drinking with friends, family, or alone?
-What was your first drink? (beer, wine?)
-How often did you drink - daily, weekly, on weekends?
-When did you drink - with friends, at parties, at home?
-Did you see an increase in your drinking?
-Did you need to drink more to get high?
-On the average, how much do you drink in one week?
-On the average, how much do you drink at one time?
-Have you ever experienced blackouts?
-Have you ever experienced craving or the need to drink?
-Have you ever experienced nausea, headaches, vomiting after drinking?
-When is the last time you had a drink? (specific day and time)
-How much did you have to drink? Where and with whom?
-Do you, or have you ever driven, after drinking?

Depending on the length of time the person admits to having an alcohol abuse history, it is wise for the counselor to recommend that the individual gets a physical examination from his/her doctor. It is important to identify any existing physical complications that may have resulted due to a chronic alcohol problem or have been exacerbated due to alcohol abuse. Since certain physical illnesses may be reversed or stopped through total alcohol abstinence, identification of such complications can result in appropriate treatment and a healthier outlook for the client.

Since the alcohol abusing individual tends to minimize the extent of their alcohol problem, the counselor should always request to speak with the individual's spouse, parent, or an individual that clearly would have knowledge of the person's alcohol use history. Requesting the presence of a person familiar with the client's alcohol history is not uncommon and in many instances standard operating procedure when seeing a client for the first time due to alcohol related problems.

In addition to gathering information pertaining to alcohol history, the counselor must also ask questions pertaining to specific drugs. Researchers have documented that individuals who abuse alcohol may also have experimented with or become addicted to various drugs.

Marijuana/pot:
   -Did you ever smoke pot?
   -How old were you? Who got you started?
   -When was the last time you smoked pot? - - How much?
   -How much money do you spend on smoking pot in a week?
   -To your knowledge has it been laced with cocaine, PCP, or any other drug?

Cocaine:
   -Did you ever try cocaine?
   -How old were you? Who got you started?
   -Did you snort? How much, how many grams per week on the average? How much money were you spending on coke?
   -Do you share straws? Do you have bleeding or perforated nasal membranes?
   -Have you smoked cocaine/crack (freebase)? How much?
   -What about IV (intravenous) use? Have you shared needles?
   -When was the last time you used cocaine?
   -What was the longest time you went between using?
   -Do you use any other drugs or drink while doing cocaine?
   -Did you use cocaine to calm or slow

down?

PCP, heroin, inhalants, valium, xanax, LSD, stimulants, depressants, etc.:
   -Please tell me about any other drugs that you have used or experimented with. When was the last time?

HIV/AIDS:
   Based on the answers to any of the preceding questions (e.g., sharing needles, sharing cocaine straws with bleeding nasal passages, unsafe sexual practices with numerous partners, either heterosexual, bisexual, or gay) the following question should be asked of the client:
   -Have you ever been HIV tested? If yes, when? what was the result - negative or positive. If negative, where you retested?
   If the counselor feels that the person may need HIV testing, the counselor must do HIV pretest counseling and an assessment of suicide risk pertaining to test outcome. The counselor must also apprise the individual that the HIV test is voluntary and is also confidential and anonymous at specific HIV test sites.

Mental Status Exam:
   The mental status exam is conducted in order for the counselor to assess the person's affect/mood, any perceptual disorders, insight and judgment, intelligence range, sleep or appetite disturbances and any possible suicide risk. The counselor at this point must assess the individual's potential to hurt either him/herself or anyone else. History pertaining to suicide attempts and/or violence toward another is important information in order to prevent future attempts and ascertain what incidents in the person's life have led to such destructive behavior(s).
   Upon completion of the comprehensive psychosocial evaluation, the counselor outlines appropriate treatment plans for the client. The treatment plan consists of type of counseling recommended for the client together

with the type of setting conducive for the client's rehabilitation from alcohol/drugs. Based on the duration and severity of the individual's alcohol problem and impact on his/her life, the client may either enter an inpatient facility for medical detoxification or agree to weekly counseling on an outpatient basis. The following section briefly summarizes the existing treatment modalities that address alcohol related problems.

II. TREATMENT MODALITIES

Today many treatment modalities exist that can assist the alcohol-abusing individual and/or his/her family members. The following are examples of the many successful treatment approaches that are available in most communities:

A. Outpatient Clinics

Outpatient services foster complete abstinence from all forms of mood-altering drugs. The purpose of the outpatient clinic is to assist the individual in dealing with his/her alcohol/drug problem while still working and functioning within the community. Within the outpatient environment the individual may attend individual and group counseling sessions, as well as education classes that teach the individual about the hazards of alcohol abuse.

In addition to receiving structured counseling time, alcohol abusing individuals are also advised to attend self-help groups, e.g., AA, (Al-Anon, ACOA for family members). The purpose of attending the self-help groups is to gain the understanding that the individual with alcohol problems can receive help and support from fellow group members. Once the person has been discharged from the outpatient clinic, he/she is well grounded in the principles of self-help groups, and he/she is often advised to continue to attend such meetings in order to maintain sobriety and prevent relapse.

B. AA, Al-Anon Self Help Groups

The Twelve Steps approach was developed by Alcoholics Anonymous (AA) as an alternative to professional counseling services. Within the AA meeting, members are welcomed unconditionally to share their histories with fellow participants. Regular attendance at AA meetings is advocated in order to maintain sobriety and prevent relapse. The self-help group also presents a forum for the recovering member to learn how other people were faced with the challenge of abstaining from alcohol and have succeeded. One of the beliefs that AA members foster is the fact that alcoholism is a physical and emotional disease rather than a question of no willpower or moral weakness. Al-Anon and ACOA are also 12-Step self-help groups for family members of alcohol abusing individual.

The Twelve Steps refer to the principles and practices that AA members espouse and practice in order to maintain and find comfort in their sobriety. AA members are not forced to adhere to these principles but merely encouraged. A list of the Twelve Steps may be obtained from any AA office.

Today, Twelve Step support groups offer groups for women, adolescents, gays/lesbians, and other personalized groups.

C. Inpatient Treatment

Inpatient treatment may be suggested if the alcohol abusing individual needs a medically supervised detoxification or has a high potential for relapse without intensive and structured supervision. A non-medical detoxification may be appropriate if the individual does not need prescribed medication. The length of time that a person may be inpatient is contingent upon the severity of the alcohol problem and high relapse factor. Within the inpatient framework, individual, family, and group counseling services are also provided. Today, many inpatient treatment programs find that the Twelve Step programs are key elements of successful, long-term recovery.

SUMMARY

Today there are several ways to assess the extent of alcohol involvement in an individual's life. One simple way is for a person to answer yes or no questions to a multi-item questionnaire to determine if in fact the person has a problem with alcohol. Based on the results of this easy to understand and easy to answer questionnaire, the person may feel that he/she needs the assistance of a qualified health professional to address his/her alcohol issues. Once the person connects with a trained alcohol counselor, the counselor may conduct a comprehensive psychosocial evaluation. This extensive evaluation process is often completed in more than one appointment. The psychosocial evaluation addresses family history, personal alcohol/drug history, educational and vocational history and a mental status exam.

Once the psychosocial evaluation is completed, the counselor together with the client determine the best treatment approach. The broad continuum of treatment approaches includes intensive inpatient rehabilitation that involves medical detoxification to less intensive weekly or biweekly counseling sessions to self-help groups such as AA. Whereas an intensive inpatient facility is often necessary for an individual with a chronic and heavy intake of alcohol, an outpatient clinic is more helpful for a person who can remain abstinent with proper support systems and continue living and working in the community.

Generally speaking, the most successful treatment approach is designed specifically to meet the needs of the individual. Any treatment approach, however, must address relapse prevention. Alcohol relapse education and prevention must be an ongoing process throughout treatment. The individual in recovery will remain successful in his/her sobriety only if he/she has been provided with information pertaining to the physical and psychosocial complications caused by alcohol use and abuse. Knowledge of support networks (e.g., AA, Al-Anon, ACOA) available in the community will also assist the individual in remaining abstinent from alcohol and ultimately prevent or halt any physical or psychosocial disabilities resulting from chronic alcohol use.

INDEX

A

AA, see Alcoholics Anonymous
Absenteeism, 77–78, 80, see also Social consequences, work environment
Abstension, 34, 35
Abuse, see also Alcoholism
  alcohol
    criteria vs. dependence, 5–6
    families, 142–143
    psychosocial evaluation, 177–178
    spinal cord injuries, 69
  drug
    alcoholics, 98–103
    homeless, 163, 164
    psychosocial evaluation, 178–179
  child, 72–75
  spouse, 72
  tobacco, 103–105
Accidents, 99, 100, see also Social consequences, accidents
Acetaldehyde, 17
ACOA, 180, 181
Acquired Immune Deficiency Syndrome (AIDS), 44–46, 179
Active coping, see Coping
Acute/chronic illness, see also Individual entries
  AIDS, 44–46
  blood disorders, 36–37
  brain, 39–43
  breast cancer, 39
  colon/rectum, 31
  endocrine system, 38
  esophagus, 30
  heart, 34–35
  hypertension and stroke, 36
  liver, 32–34
  mouth, 29–30
  musculoskeletal system, 35–36
  pancreas, 31–32
  pulmonary disease, 37–38
  seizures, 43
  sexual dysfunction, 38–39
  stomach and small intestine, 30–31
ADA, see Americans With Disabilities Act of 1990
Adaptability in families, 150–151, see also Families, alcoholism
Addiction, 69, see also Abuse, drug
Adolescents, 100–101, 102, 112, see also Teenagers
Adrenal glands, 117
African Americans, 19, 71
Age, 40–41, 60
Aggression, 73, 142, see also Antisocial behavior
Aging, 121, see also Nutrition
Agnosia, 43
AIDS, see Acquired Immune Deficiency Syndrome
Al-Alon, 180, 181
Albumin, 118, see also Nutrition
Alcohol abuse, see Abuse, alcohol
Alcohol Amnestic Disorder, see Korsakoff's Psychosis
Alcohol assessment tools
  psychosocial evaluation
    alcohol/drug history, 176–178
    educational and vocational history, 174–175
    HIV/AIDS, 179
    legal history, 176
    marijuana history, 178–179
    mental status, 179–180
    military history, 175–176
    personal and family history, 172–174
    presenting problem, 170–171
    previous treatment, 171–172
    treatment modalities, 180–182
    use questionaire, 169–170
Alcoholic beverages usage, 93
Alcoholic disability, 1, 2–3
Alcoholics Anonymous, 180, 181, see also Self-help groups
Alcoholism
  definition, 1–2
  family, see Family, alcoholism
  historical perspective, 11
  overview, 93–95
  prevalence, 6–7
  stages of drinking, 95–98
ALMACA, see Association of Labor Management Administrators and Consultants on Alcoholism

Alzheimer's Disease, 43
Amblyopia, 117
Amenorrhea, 39
American Medical Society on Alcoholism (AMSA), 94
Americans With Disabilities Act of 1990 (ADA), 1
Amino acids, 116, 117, 122–123, see also Nutrition
Amnesia, psychogenic, 73, 143
Amphetamines, 99, 100, see also Abuse, drug
AMSA, see American Medical Society on Alcoholism
Anemia, see also Homelessness; Nutrition
  alcohol relation, 36
  homeless, 165
  nutritional relation, 115, 116, 117, 119
Anesthetics, 66, 99
Anorexia, 121, see also Nutrition
Antidepressants, 102, see also Abuse, drug
Antihistamines, 99
Antisocial behavior, 101, 102, 142, 163, 164
Anxiety, 3, 141–142, see also Family, alcoholism
Aphasia, 66
Appetite, 116, see also Nutrition
Apraxia, 43
Arrhythmia, 34, see also Heart
Assessment, ass Alcohol assessment tools
Association of Labor-Management Administrators and Consultants on Alcoholism (ALMACA), 76, 79
Attention span, 21, 65

B

BAC, see Blood alcohol concentration
Balance, loss of, 63, see also Social consequences, accidents
BALs, see Blood alcohol levels
Barbiturates, 99, 100, see also Abuse, drug
Behavior, development, 21
Benzodiazepines, 99
Beriberi, 116
Bile, 32
Birth defects, 15–20, 121
Blackout, 40
Bladder, 68
Bleeding, 32, 114, 115, 119, see also Hemorrhage; Nutrition

Blisters, 37
Blood, 36–37, see also Red blood cells
Blood alcohol concentration (BAC), 59–60, 63, 64, 96
Blood alcohol levels (BALs), 15, 164
Blood-brain barrier, 15
Blood clotting, 36, 114
Blood pressure, 37, see also Hypertension
Blood sugar, 32, 36, 38, 123
Blood vessels, 115, see also Nutrition
Boating, 62–63, see also Social consequences, accidents
Body heat, 63
Body length of fetus, 17, see also Fetal Alcohol Syndrome
Bone marrow, 44–45, 115, 117, see also Nutrition
Bones, 36, 113, 115, 118, see also Nutrition
Boredom, 67–68
Bowel, 68
Brain, 15, 32, 39–43, 124, see also Acute/chronic illness
Breast feeding, 21
Bullous, 37
Burns, 63–64, see also Social consequences, accidents

C

Caffeine, 103
Calcium, 113, 118–119, see also Nutrition
Cancer, see also Acute/chronic illness
  breast, 39
  esophogus, 30
  liver, 34
  oral, 29, 104
  pancreatis, 32
  stomach, 31
Carbohydrate metabolism, 115–117, see also Nutrition
Cardiac arrest, 120, see also Heart, disorders and nutrition
Cardiomyopathy, 35, see also Heart, disorders and nutrition
Cardiovascular disorders, 162, 163, 165, see also Homelessness
Caucasians, 19
Cell damage, 113–114, see also Nutrition
Center for Disease Control, 112
Center for Environmental Health, 64
Central nervous system (CNS), 16, 20, 66, 99, 120, see also Brain

Index

Chaotic family systems, 150–152, see also Family, alcoholism
Child abuse, see Abuse, child
Children of alcoholic families, 141–142, see also Family, alcoholism
Cholesterol, 124, 125, see also Nutrition
Cigarettes, 63–64, see also Social consequences, accidents
Cirrhosis, 33–34, 119, see also Liver
CNS, see Central nervous system
Cocaine, 44, 99, 100, 101, see also Abuse, drug
Code of Hammurabi, 11
Coenzymes, 114–117
Cognitive functioning, 40–41, 67
Cohension, 150
Colon, 31, see also Acute/chronic illness
Colorectal cancer, 31, see also Cancer
Coma, 66, 99, 124
Communication, 140–141, see also Family, alcoholism
Community for Creative Non-Violence, 161
Conception, 18
Condoms, see Contraceptives
Conduct problems, 142, see also Antisocial behavior
Confabulation, 65
Congestive heart failure, 35, see also Heart
Connective tissue, 115
Contraceptives, 46
Coping with stress, 145–153
Coronary artery disease, 125
Counseling, 68, 146–147, 171–172, see also Alcohol assessment tools
Crime, 69–70, 101, see also Social consequences
Crisis, 146
Cross-tolerance, 99
Crying, 73, see also Abuse, child
C. Everett Koop, 22

D

Deliquency, 101, 102, see also Antisocial behavior
Dementia, 42–43, see also Mental disorders
Denial, 147, see also Family, alcoholism
Deoxyribonucleic acid (DNA), 15
Depression, 3, 115, 116, 141, 142, see also Family, alcoholism
Dermatitis, 117
Detoxification, 165

Diabetes, 38
Diagnosis, 3–4, see also Alcohol assessment tools
Diagnostic and Statistical Manual of Mental Disorders (DSM), 5–6, 41–42, 75, 96–98, 163
Disease concept, 95, see also Alcoholism
Disengaged family system, 150, see also Family, alcoholism
Distress, 73, 142, see also Abuse, child
Diving reflex, 63
Divorce, 72
DNA, see Deoxyribonucleic acid
Dosage, alcohol, 35
Driving while intoxicated (DWI), 95, 96, see also Drunken driving
Drowning, 62–63, see also Social consequences, accidents
Drug abuse, see Abuse, drug
Drunken driving, 59–61
DSM, see Diagnostic and Statistical Manual of Mental Disorders
Duodenum, 30–31
DWI, see Driving while intoxicated
Dysarthria, 66
Dysfunction cycle, 148, 149

E

EAP Coordinator, 78
Earnings, 4–5
Education, 41, 68, 174–175
Emergency shelters, 161, 164, 165–166
Emotional bonding, 150, see also Family, alcoholism
Emotional development, 141, see also Family, alcoholism
Emotional distress, 147, 163, see also Family, alcoholism
Employee Assistance Professionals Association (EAPA), 76, 79
Employee Assistance Programs (EAPs), 79–80
Encephalopathy, 43, see also Brain
Endocarditis, 34, see also Heart
Endocrine system, 38, see also Acute/chronic illness
Energy, production, 116, 117, 120, see also Nutrition
Enlarged heart, 35, see also Heart
Enmeshed family system, 150–152, see also Family, alcoholism

Epilepsy, 43, see also Seizure disorders
Esophagitis, 30, 119
Esophagus, 30, see also Acute/chronic illness
Estrogen, excess production in males, 39
Estropia, 16
Ethanol, 29–30

F

Facial dysmorphology, 16
FAE, see Fetal alcohol effects
Falls, 64, see also Social consequences, accidents
Family
  alcoholism
    alcoholic children, 139–141
    emotional effects on offspring, 141–142
    familial, 65, 67
    overview, 137–138
    stress, 143–153
    summary, 153
    violence, 142–143
  history, 172–174
  secrets, 151
  violence, 71–72
FAS, see Fetal Alcohol Syndrome
Fat, 115, 124–126, see also Nutrition
Fatalities, 59, 60, 63–64, see also Social consequences, accidents
Fatigue, 116
Fatty acids, 117, 124–126, see also Nutrition
Fatty liver, 33
Federal Railroad Administration, 78
Feeding, 21
Fertility, 38
Fetal alcohol effects (FAE), 17–19, see also Fetal Alcohol Syndrome
Fetal Alcohol Syndrome (FAS)
  characterization, 15–20
  glucose levels, 124
  smoking and alcohol relation, 103–104
  zinc deficiency, 121
Fetus, 15–22, see also Fetal Alcohol Syndrome
Fibrillation, 34, see also Heart
Fight/flight response, 146
Fires, 63–64, see also Social consequences, accidents
Flying, 61–62, see also Social consequences, accidents

Folate, 36, 117–118, see also Nutrition
Food, see also Nutrition
  mineral sources, 117–121
  vitamin sources, 112–117
Frontal lobe, 67

G

Gastritis, 30, 94, 119
Gastrointestinal disorders, 162, 163, 164, see also Gastritis
Gender
  alcohol abuse vs. dependence, 6–7
  boating accidents, 63
  child abuse, 73
  homelessness, 163
  risk of becoming alcoholic, 139, 140
  sexual dysfunction, 38–39
  smoking, 103
  traffic-related accidents, 60
Genetics, 139–140
Glucose, 17, 123–124
Glycogen, 123
Goal setting, unrealistic, 66
Growth, 15, 20, 120, 124, see also Fetal Alcohol Syndrome; Nutrition

H

Hair loss, 120
Hallucinosis, 41
Harris Poll, 1
HDL, see High density lipoprotein
Head injuries, 4, 64–68, see also Social consequences, accidents
Head size, 18
Health care, 80, 161–162, see also Homelessness
Hearing disorders, 16
Heart
  acute/chronic illness, 34–35
  disorders and nutrition, 116, 118, 120, 121, 125
  fetal, 18
Hemoglobin, 119
Hemorrhage, 30, 66, 114
Hepatic encephalopathy, 122, see also Liver
Hepatitis, 33, 121, see also Liver
Heroin, 100, see also Abuse, drug
High density lipoprotein (HDL), 125
Hip, 36
HIV, see Human immunodeficiency virus
Homelessness, 161–166

Index

Hormone production, 117
Human immunodeficiency virus (HIV), 44–46, 179
Hyperactivity, 16, see also Fetal Alcohol Syndrome
Hyperglycemia, 123–124, see also Blood sugar
Hyperlipidemia, 36–37. 124, 125
Hypertension, 37, 162, 163
Hypocalcemia, 118
Hypoglycemia, 36, 38. 123–124, see also Blood sugar
Hypogonadism, 121
Hypomagnesemia, 120

I

Immune system, 44–46, 121
Infection, post-injury, 67
Inflammation, 116, 120
Injuries, traffic accidents, 59–60, see also Social consequences, accidents
Inmates, 70, see also Social consequences, crime and violence
Inpatient treatment, 181–182, see also Alcohol assessment tools
Insulin, 120
Intoxication, 41, 60–61, see also Individual entries
Intrauterine growth retardation (IUGR), 104
IQ, 19, see also Fetal Alcohol Syndrome
Iron, 115, 119, see also Nutrition
IUGR, see Intrauterine growth retardation

J

Jaundice, 33, 34, see also Liver
Judgment, impaired, 43, 67

K

Kaposi's Sarcoma, 45, see also Acquired Immune Deficiency Syndrome
Ketosis, 38
Kidney, 32, 35, 120
Korsakoff's Psychosis, 41–42

L

Lactate dehydrogenase, 165
Lactic acidosis, 38
Larynx, 104, 105, see also Cancer
LBW, see Low birth weight

Learning disabilities, 17, 19, 40, see also Fetal Alcohol Syndrome
Legal history, 176, see also Alcohol assessment tools
Lesions, 40, see also Brain
Librium, 99, see also Abuse, drugs
Lipids, 124–126, see also Nutrition
Liver
  acute/chronic illness of, 32–34
  enzymes, 165
  homelessness, 162, 164
  nutritional deficiency, 111, 113, 114, 121, 124–125
Low birth weight (LBW), 20–21
Lung disease, 37–38, 162, 163, 164, 165

M

Magnesium, 119–120, see also Nutrition
Malabsorption, 118, see also Nutrition
Mallory-Weiss syndrome, 30
Malnutrition, 31, 165, see also Homelessness
Mammary glands, 39
Manslaughter, 70, see also Social consequences, crime and violence
Marijuana, 99, 100, 101, see also Abuse, drug
MCV, see Mean corpuscular volume
Mean corpuscular hemoglobin, 165
Mean corpuscular volume (MCV), 36
Medical training, 4
Memory impairment, 40, 41, 65, 115, 116
Menstruation, 39
Mental disorders, 141, 163–164
Mental retardation, 15, 16, see also Fetal Alcohol Syndrome
Metabolism, 32, 111, 115, 116, 117
Microencephaly, 17, see also Fetal Alcohol Syndrome
Midbrain, 67
Military history evaluation, 175–176
Minerals, 31, 118–122, see also Nutrition
Miscarriage, 17
Mood swings, 65
Morality, 33
Morphine, 100, see also Abuse, drug
Morphogenesis of family units, 146, see also Family, alcoholism
Mortality statistics, 20, 99
Motor dysfunction, 40
Motorcycles, 60, see also Social consequences, accidents

Mouth, 29–30, 117, see also Acute/chronic illness; Nutrition
Mouthwash, 29–30
Mucous membranes, 30
Multiplicative hypothesis, 104–105
Murder, 70, see also Social consequences, crime and violence
Muscles
  breast milk, 21
  damage and alcohol, 35
  nutrition relation, 114, 119, 120, 121
Musculoskeletal system, 35–36, see also Acute/chronic illness
Myopathy, 35–36

N

Nasal bridge, 17
NASS, see National Accident Sampling System
National Accident Sampling System (NASS), 59–60
National Cancer Institute, 39, 105
National Census for Health Statistics, 1, 5
National Council on Alcoholism (NCA), 62, 94
National Council on Alcoholism and Drug Dependence (NCADD), 2
National Head Injury Foundation, 65–66
National Health Interview Survey (NHIS), 1
National Highway Traffic Safety Administration, 59
National Institute on Alcohol Abuse, 62
National Institute on Alcohol Abuse and Alcoholism (NIAAA), 5, 31
National Institute on Drug Abuse, 98–99, 100
NCA, see National Council on Alcoholism
NCADD, see National Council on Alcoholism and Drug Dependence
Nembutal, 99, see also Abuse, drug
Nervous system, 115, see also Nutrition
Neurological disorders, 114, 165, see also Homelessness; Nutrition
New York State Division of Alcohol and Alcohol Abuse, 44
NHIS, see National Health Interview Survey
NIAAA, see National Institute on Alcohol Abuse and Alcoholism
Night driving, 59, see also Social consequences, accidents
Night vision, 113, 121

Nonnormative stressors, 145, see also Coping
Normative stressors, 145, see also Coping
Nucleic acids, 117, 120
Nursing infants, 21–22
Nutrient absorption, 31
Nutrition
  amino acids, 122–123
  glucose, 123–124
  lipids, fats, and fatty acids, 124–126
  minerals, 118–122
  overview, 111–112
  summary, 126–128
  vitamins, 112–118
Nystagmus, 42

O

Optic nerve hypoplasia, 16, see also Fetal Alcohol Syndrome
Oral/motor impairment, 65, see also Social consequences, accidents
Oropharynx, 104, 105
Orthopedic disabilities, 102, see also Abuse, drug
Osteonecrosis, idiopathic, 36
Osteopemia, 36
Osteoporosis, 36, 113, see also Bones
Outdoor living, 165–166, see also Homelessness
Outpatient clinics, 180–181, see also Alcohol assessment tools
Oxygen, 17, 62, 121

P

Palliative coping, see Coping
Pancreas, 31–32, see also Acute/chronic illness
Pancreatitis, 32
Paranoia, 71
Paraplegia, 68
PCP, see Phenylcyclidine
Perception, 40, 67
Perinatal period, 20–22
Pernicious anemia, 115, see also Anemia
Personality, 65, 141
Phenylcyclidine (PCP), 100
Phosphate, 113
Phospholipids, 124
Photophobia, 117
Pilots, 61–62, see also Social consequences, accidents

Index

Placenta, 15, 20
Platelets, 36
PMNs, see Polymorphonuclear leukocytes
Pneumatoceles, 37
Pneumocystic carinii pneumonia, 45, see also Acquired Immune Deficiency Syndrome
Pneumonia, 37, see also Lung disease
Polymorphonuclear leukocytes (PMNs), 44–45
Portal-systemic encephalopathy (PSE), 122
Post-traumatic stress disorder, 73–74, 142–143, see also Coping
Pregnancy, 15, 124
Prescription drugs, 102, see also Abuse, drug
Prevention of alcohol abuse, 7–8
Primary malnutrition, 111, 113, 114, see also Nutrition
Problem solving, 16, 137, 138, 152, see also Coping
Prostaglandins, 121
Proteins, 31, 120
Psychedelic drugs, 100, see also Abuse, drug
Psychoactive substance abuse, 98
Psychoactive substance dependence, 97
Psychogenic amnesia, see Amnesia, psychogenic
Pubic hair, 39
Pulmonary disease, see Lung disease
Pyridoxone, see Vitamin B6

Q

Quadriplegia, 68

R

Rape, 70–71, see also Social consequences, crime and violence
Rats, 19–20
RBCs, see Red blood cells
Rearing practices, 140
Reasoning, abstract, 65
Recidivism, 67–68
Recovery from head injuries, 66, 67, see also Social consequences, accidents
Rectum, 31, see also Acute/chronic illness
Red blood cells (RBCs)
   elimination by reticuloendothelial system, 45
   formation, 36
   vitamin role, 113–114, 115, 117
Responsibilities, 147–148
Reticuloendothelial system, 45
Retina, 16, see also Fetal Alcohol Syndrome
Riboflavin, 36, 117, see also Nutrition
Rickets, 113, see also Nutrition
Rigid family systems, 151–152, see also Family, alcoholism
Risk, alcoholism in children, 139
Risk-taking, 61, 62–63, see also Social consequences, accidents
Role reversal, 147–148, 149, 150, 152, see also Family, alcoholism
Rules, 150–151

S

Scar tissue, 34
Schizophrenia, 41
School-age children, 18
SCI, see Spinal cord injury
Scurvy, 115, see also Nutrition
Seconal, 99, see also Abuse, drug
Secondary malnutrition, 111, 113, see also Nutrition
Sedative drugs, 95, see also Abuse, drugs
Sedative-hypnotic drugs, 99, see also Abuse, drugs
Seizure disorders, 43, 162, 164, see also Homelessness
Selenium, 121–122, see also Nutrition
Self-esteem, 153
Self-help groups, 146–147, 180, 181
Sensory perception, 66
Serotonin, 122
Serum urea nitrogen, 165
Sexual assault, 70–71, see also Social consequences, crime and violence
Sexual dysfunction, 38–39, 68, 113
Sexually transmitted disease, 45–46, 165, see also Homelessness
Skin disorders, 116, 120, see also Nutrition
Sleep disorders, 16, 21, 116
Small intestine, 30–31, see also Acute/chronic illness; Gastrointestinal disorders
Smoking, 21, 29, 30, see also Cancer; Abuse, tobacco
Social consequences
   accidents
      boating and drownings, 62–63
      falls, 64

fires and burns, 63–64
flying, 61–62
head injuries, 64–68
spinal cord injuries, 68–69
traffic, 59–61
crime and violence
family, 71–75
overview, 69–71
summary, 81–83
work environment
dealing with abuse, 79–81
other consequences, 78–79
overview, 75–77
tardiness and absenteeism, 77–78
Speech disorders, 16, see also Fetal Alcohol Syndrome
Spinal cord injury (SCI), 4, 68–69, see also Social consequences, accidents
Spouse abuse, see Abuse, spouse
Stillbirth, 15
Stomach, 30–31, see also Acute/chronic illness; Gastrointestinal disorders
Strabismus, 16
Stress, 65, 140, 143–153
Stroke, 37, 125
Support groups, see Self-help groups
Swimming, 63
Synergism, 99, 104–105

T

T lymphocytes, 45
Tardiness, 77–78, see also Social consequences, work environments
Teenagers, 61, 71, see also Adolescents
Teeth, 113, 115, 118, see also Nutrition
Temperature, body, 120
Testicles, atrophy, 38
Testosterone, 38
Thiamin, 42, 116–117, see also Nutrition
Tinnitus, 66
Tissue, elasticity, 121, see also Nutrition
Tobacco abuse, see Abuse, tobacco
Tongue, 104, 117, see also Cancer
Toxin accumulation, 17, 34, see also Fetal Alcohol Syndrome
Toxoplasmosis, 45
Tranquilizers, 99, see also Abuse, drug
Trauma, 162, 164, see also Homelessness
Treatment, 96, 98, 180–182
Triglycerides, 124, 125
Tryptophan, 122–123

Twelve steps approach, 181, see also Self-help groups
Twins, 140

U

Ulcers, 30–31, 119, see also Gastritis; Gastrointestinal disorders
United States, alcohol usage statistics, 93
United States Bureau of Census, 161
United States Coast Guard, 62
United States Department of Health and Human Resources, 72–73
United States Department of Health and Human Services, 59
United States Department of Housing and Urban Development, 161
United States Department of Justice, 70
United States Surgeon General, 22
Urine, 38, 121

V

Vaginal bleeding, 20, see also Bleeding; Hemorrhage
Valium, 99, 100, see also Abuse, drug
Vasculature, retina, 16
Victims of violence, 73–74, 142–143, see also Family, alcoholism; Social consequences, crime and violence
Violence, see Social consequences, crime and violence
Vision disorders, 16
Vitamin A, 112–113
Vitamin B1, see Thiamin
Vitamin B12, 115
Vitamin B2, see Riboflavin
Vitamin B6, 116
Vitamin C, 115
Vitamin D, 113
Vitamin E, 113–114
Vitamin K, 36, 114
Vitamins, see also Nutrition
absorption in stomach and small intestine, 31
deficiency and oral cancer, 29
fat-soluble, 112–114
water-soluble, 114–118
Vocational history evaluation, 174–175, see also Alcohol assessment tools

W

War on Drugs, 7

WBCs, see White blood cells
Wernicke-Korsakoff Syndrome, 42, 116
White blood cells (WBCs), 37, see also Blood; Red blood cells
Witness to violence, 73–74, 142–143, see also Family, alcoholism; Social consequences, crime and violence

Work environment, 75–77, see also Social consequences
Work quality, 78
Wound healing, 115, 120, see also Nutrition

Z

Zinc, 29, 120–121, see also Nutrition